BURAK M OZGUR MD

GRABBING LIFE *by the* HORNS

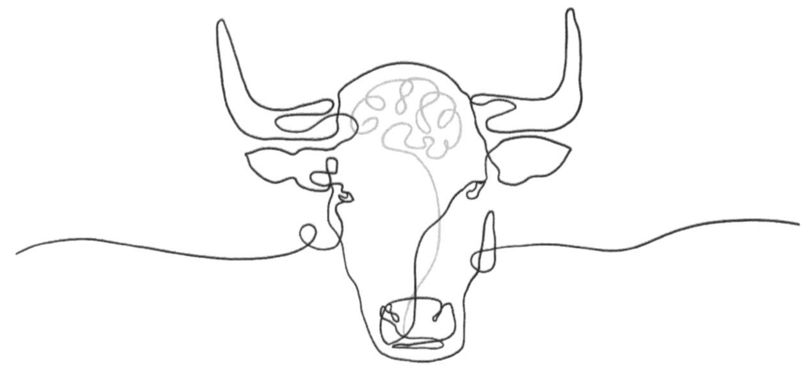

AND OTHER PATIENT STORIES OF A NEUROSURGEON

Grabbing Life By The Horns and Other Patient Stories of a Neurosurgeon By Burak M Ozgur, MD
Published 2022 by Your Book Angel

ozgurmd.com
Instagram @burakozgurmd

Printed in the United States
Edited by Keidi Keating
Layout by Rochelle Mensidor

Cover and Illustrations by Hala Khalifeh at Halaballoo
https://halaballoo.shop/
Instagram @halaballoo.shop

ISBN: 979-8-9850627-5-5

Table of Contents

Introduction

Life is a beautiful and miraculous gift! I feel that I have a unique perspective on life due to the fact that I have the honor to serve as a neurosurgeon. It is such a blessing to be able to help fellow human beings in their time of need, their struggle for quality of life, and sometimes for life itself. Where else do you have someone say to you, "...go ahead and put me to sleep and while my eyes are closed, take a knife and cut me. Perform surgery on my brain or spine, and I TRUST you to try and make me better..." There is an immeasurable trust indeed put into us as neurosurgeons to help. I don't take that honor or trust lightly.

I learned so much from my parents. My mother dedicated her life to life-long learning and educating others. Teachers are so underappreciated when in fact they are the backbone of our youngest generation in their most formative years. They should be among our most honored in society. I learned from my mother to value education and learning from every experience. She taught me to take advantage and invest in all learning opportunities. This investment would indeed pay dividends in the future. My father is a retired neurosurgeon. He is the humblest man I know. Even now, he still drives a minivan. Why would he do this when all the kids are grown and moved out? It's because he has always valued time spent together. Whenever we visit, if we go out, he finds value in the precious moments driving somewhere together. If you ever saw him walking around or shopping at Costco, you would have no idea what he does for a living because he's always dressed so modestly. He values every profession and always says that no person is better than another just because they may have been blessed with money, education, or other opportunities. He'd say teachers, janitors, doctors, nurses, and gardeners are all important and provide important services to society. He would always instill in my siblings and me the warning not to be arrogant. Growing up, I remember that he never gave a hard time to patients who couldn't pay for his services. Some of his most prized "payments for services" were knitted scarves from a nun, or a box of oranges from a farmer. He was always grateful for what he had and what he could provide to others. My father also taught me to learn from every experience. As physicians, we always try our best, but despite that, we may sometimes have complications. We should always strive to learn from our successes but even more from our failures, or complications, and those of others so as not to repeat them.

The journey to becoming a neurosurgeon is a long, arduous, fifteen-year-long ultra-marathon. This path would have been impossible without the love and support of my family. I thank them for putting up with me through all the years. My wonderful, loving, supportive, and patient wife has been there from the beginning, and every step of the way. She deserves the degree just as much as I, for I could not have done any of it without her. We had our kids during this journey. Our first son was born during my gross anatomy class in medical school. Our second son was born during my ob-gyn rotation. Our daughter was born during residency. They all made sacrifices for all the times I was in the hospital on-call and couldn't be at home with them. I will never forget the day that my wife offered to take them to Disneyland but the kids instead chose to come to the hospital and have lunch with me since I was again on-call that weekend. They all sacrificed for my chosen profession, so I made my best attempt to always be there for them every minute that I was home. I remember once finding my younger son asleep on the floor in front of the front door of our apartment when I was a neurosurgery resident. Beside him was a little Lego structure that he had built. When I asked him what he had made, he said he had built a hospital so that I could work from home and didn't have to leave. It's experiences like these that would bring tears to my eyes but would also ensure that I wouldn't take anything for granted. I would always work hard to try and be the best I could be at everything. My wife could tell you that sometimes I beat myself up too much if things aren't perfect. I honestly want the best outcome for each and every patient. Although sometimes things may not turn out that way, I stay up late and study each case and try to learn what I could have done differently. I do all this because of both the sacrifices so many of my family members and friends have made to help get me here, and out of honor and respect for the trust patients bestow on me. I can never take any of that for granted.

As a neurosurgeon, I am always conscious of the need for balance between clinical detachment and empathy. Being able to provide objective, unbiased care while inspiring trust and confidence in my patients is a skill I have developed over the course of my career as a neurosurgeon. At the core of every good doctor there remains an unwavering desire to help others. I see patients in their most vulnerable moments—often at a time when their life, or their quality of life, hangs in the balance. I am constantly humbled and grateful for the trust my patients and their families place in me, and I strive every day to be worthy of that honor.

As a child, I loved working with my hands. I was constantly taking things apart, much to my parents' chagrin. Be it a bike, a radio, or whatever else I could get my hands on, I felt this deep-seated pull to understand the mechanics of how things worked. I suppose it makes sense that I would choose a profession that allows me to work with my hands every day. When I first began my medical studies, I was drawn to neuroscience because so much about it is still a mystery. I like to compare the human brain to space in the sense that there is still so much to explore and discover. If you look back on what we knew about the human brain twenty, or even ten years ago, so much of our understanding has changed. New evidence and data continues to challenge what we thought we knew, and we are all the better for it. I am constantly learning from my patients, and I use the knowledge I acquire from each new case to help other patients.

While highly skilled in their domain, doctors are still human beings with feelings and emotions just like anyone else. Many of the cases I see stay with me long after a patient case has been closed. In many ways, they become like family while they are under my care, and I treat them with the same compassion, respect, and dedication that I would if we were related by blood. At the end of the day, I may take home feelings of satisfaction, joy, disappointment, or sorrow, but always I am left with a sense of wonder at the juxtaposition between fragility and tenacity of the human body.

I decided to share with you this collection of stories from some of my most memorable and interesting case files. Some of the stories may seem miraculous, others tragic, but they are all unique and inspiring in their own way. In his book "The Man Who Mistook his Wife for a Hat," famed neurologist Oliver Sacks observes, "With the rise of neuroscience and all its wonders, it is even more important now to preserve the personal narrative, to see each patient as a unique being with [their] own history and strategies for adapting and surviving."

I feel blessed every day to be able to do the work that I do, and to be able to help people in their time of need. It is through the collective experiences of my patients that I witness the fascinating complexity and undiscovered potential of the human brain.

The names, ages, and any identifying characteristics within these stories have been changed in order to protect the identity and privacy of the actual patients and their families.

CHAPTER 1

The Shrek Phenomenon

◇◈◆◈◆◈◇

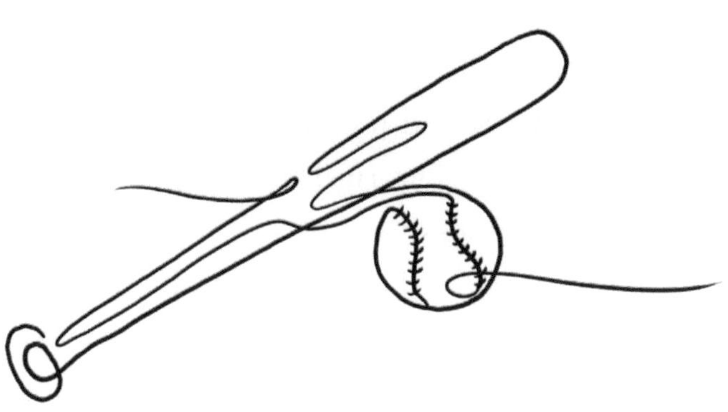

When an aspiring doctor first graduates from medical school, they have the opportunity to practice medicine in a hospital setting under the supervision of more experienced staff. As a surgical intern, each doctor-in-training must complete various rotations in many medical and surgical specialties to gain experience in, and enhance their knowledge of, the many different aspects of medicine. As a resident I was constantly expanding my understanding of the link between the human body and brain and learning to connect more effectively with my patients.

I was on call for neurosurgery at the Children's Hospital in San Diego when I first met Shawn, a happy seven-year-old boy with a shock of curly brown hair. Shawn had been brought into the emergency room by his parents out of an abundance of caution after he was struck in the head by a wayward ball at his weekly softball game. He'd complained to his parents about having a headache and feeling a little nauseous, so naturally they were concerned he may have sustained some sort of head trauma.

I performed a thorough examination and ran some tests, which included a computed axial tomography (CAT) scan to check for signs of skull or brain injury. When the results came back, the news was not good. Although the imaging showed Shawn did not have any internal hemorrhaging, fractures, or other softball-related injury, it indicated he had a large tumor at the back lower portion of his brain, which is called the cerebellum. Had Shawn not been brought in that day, the tumor would have gone undetected and continued to grow in size, leading to more serious and dangerous symptoms that would have landed him in my emergency room eventually. As a doctor, I knew how lucky it was that the tumor had been detected so early, but it also meant Shawn was going to need surgery. Further, once the tumor was removed, we'd need to have it analyzed to know whether it was cancerous. If it was, Shawn would need to undergo further treatment including radiation and chemotherapy. I was now faced with the unenviable task of breaking the news to his anxious parents.

Shawn's parents were devastated, but also supportive of the additional tests and surgery we recommended by way of next steps. Having a plan always helps to make a big problem seem more manageable, and Shawn's family was looking to me for answers and guidance. I was moved by their faith in me and resolved to do everything I could to help their little boy. Shawn was very brave and cooperative over the next few days as he underwent further tests. My colleagues and I needed to ascertain the exact location, size, and other details of the tumor before we could remove it. We determined the tumor was about the size of a golf ball. Shawn did his best to look on the bright side of things. "Maybe nonna will bring a cannoli for me to eat when I wake up," he said drowsily to his parents just before the surgery. "I love her cannoli," he added, looking at me.

The surgery took about five hours to complete, and it was a success. The tumor had been located in the cerebellum, which is an area of the brain that controls coordination and balance. His parents were overjoyed when I told them everything had gone well, and they couldn't wait to see him. When Shawn woke up after the surgery, he looked normal, but it soon became evident that all was not well. Although he could look at us, walk unassisted, move all his limbs, and could understand everything we said and take direction, he had lost his ability to speak.

His parents were dismayed, and I was perplexed. Although there are risks associated with any surgery, the area of the brain where the tumor had been located was not known to have a predominant role in the production of speech. I started combing through old textbooks and pouring through research material to find anything that might explain why this was happening. Although I did come across a few vague references, there was nothing I could find that would help my patient recover his ability to speak.

Shawn and his family were soon hit with more bad news; the pathology on his tumor came in, indicating that it was a medulloblastoma—meaning cancer. Over the next several weeks Shawn underwent treatment, and during that time, I continued to monitor his recovery on a daily basis. At the same time, I continued my search for anything that would help Shawn regain his ability to speak. During this time, I developed a close bond with his family, who came to visit him often. I came to know some of his extended family members as well, including his nonna, who, I would happily discover firsthand, was an outstanding cook. (I had the chance to sample his nonna's famed cannoli on more than one occasion—and let me tell you, they were as good as Shawn said!)

One day, while Shawn and his older sister Myra were sitting on his bed engrossed in a movie, something unusual happened. The kids were watching *Shrek*, as their parents and I chatted and observed them quietly from the hall. When it came to the part where the song "I'm a Believer," began playing, Shawn started to sing along. We watched him in disbelief until the song ended, at which time he fell silent again. Curiosity and clinical interest getting the better of me, I ran to the bed and used the TV remote to replay the song. Sure enough, as soon as the song began, Shawn started singing again. When I would pause the song, he would stop singing. We ended up playing the song over and over, and each time, Shawn happily sang along. At first, he could only vocalize when singing, but over the next several weeks and months, Shawn would regain full control of speech again, much to the relief of his family and his doctors. He also completed his cancer therapy, and I am pleased to report he has remained healthy.

That day when Shawn started singing stuck in my mind. Although I could find no documented rationale that would explain it, I began to formulate my own theory about why I thought it had happened from a mechanical perspective. The cerebellum coordinates movement, but I theorized it could also coordinate the movement of the mouth and vocalization as well, and this function may have been altered as a result of swelling on the brain from the surgery. I wrote a paper about it, wherein I touched on the different types of speech, including melodic speech and monotonal speech and suggested the link between the function of the cerebellum and other parts of the brain. Post-surgical swelling would have put pressure on the area, causing cerebellar mutism. Once the swelling from surgery went down and Shawn healed, the song from *Shrek* triggered a "restart" of his speech coordination, which first manifested in his ability to use melodic speech (also known as singing). I theorized that in addition to the well-known classical areas of the brain, there must be other areas and pathways that we have yet to fully understand. It may be that the healthy areas may help recover or "re-wire" the injured areas, as is the case when people have strokes or traumatic injury. My paper was published in a medical journal, and later picked up by *Discover* magazine.

Over the course of the next several weeks and months, letters began to pour in from all over the world. People were writing to tell me about their experiences, which were similar to this phenomenon. They were excited to understand finally, at least partially what was going on and have something to compare their experiences with.

One woman wrote to tell me of her husband's inability to speak following a stroke he suffered several years ago. She shared that although her husband could not talk, he would sing with the radio sometimes when they were in the car together. She wondered if I had any ideas about how to help him. In response, I suggested she try something a little unconventional. I explained the different types of speech to her and said perhaps her husband's ability to vocalize using melodic speech might still be possible. I recommended she try accessing his speech with more singing. In a nutshell, I told her to pretend her life was a musical, and when she started a conversation with her husband, to sing to him rather than speaking the words. As ridiculous as it may have sounded, it actually worked! She wrote back a short time later to share her excitement.

Another letter I received was from a woman who did folk singing in Florida. She volunteered every week at a nursing home, singing to the residents. Each week there would be a group of older men who had all suffered strokes and who, according to the nursing home staff, could no longer speak. She found that when she would sing a selection of old war-time songs, some of the gentlemen would begin to sing. The nursing home staff were surprised, and no one had been able to offer her an explanation. She told me when she read about my theory, everything had finally made sense.

Shawn's story has advanced our understanding of brain function and reminded us that there is still so much about the brain that we don't fully understand. The telling of his story has helped many people all around the world.

CHAPTER 2

Mother Tongue

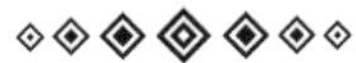

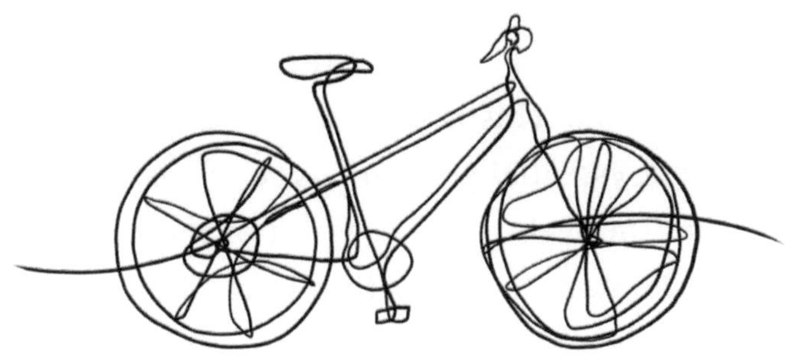

This story is about a man in his thirties named Youssef, who was hit by a car while bicycling home from work one afternoon. He was in rough shape when he was brought into the hospital, and his chances of survival were slim. He had sustained a terrible brain injury after hitting his head on the pavement. He had not been wearing a helmet at the time, and the impact to his skull had caused major brain injury and swelling. This was a problem because there is very little space between the brain and the skull, so the brain does not have much room to expand. When this sort of injury occurs, it's necessary to relieve the pressure, if the patient is to have any chance of survival.

There are several methods we use to try and bring down the pressure. We had exhausted all the standard methods and had to resort to a last effort to save his life. In this type of situation we performed a procedure that involved removing a large portion of skull to give the brain more room for expansion. This may be a little gruesome for some, but essentially, in this type of surgery you open up the scalp, then saw part of the skull off. Under the skull there is a thin layer of protection covering the brain called the dura. You make slits in the dura so it releases some of the pressure on the brain. This is a last-ditch effort to potentially save someone's life. It could be weeks before it's clear if the patient would survive and then you could replace or reconstruct the skull.

I was a neurosurgery resident when Youssef arrived at the hospital. I was working in a different rotation when Youssef was brought to the neurosurgical service, so I was not involved with his initial treatment or care. Against the odds, Youssef had survived the brain swelling and surgery, but had been in a coma for quite some time. Typically, if patients who survive this type of injury and surgery are going to recover, they regain consciousness within days or a couple of weeks. Youssef had been in a vegetative state on the neurosurgical service for about four weeks by the time I took over his case. When rotating to a new service, the resident physicians will give a debrief of their patients and sign over care. I was provided with a summary of Youssef's injury and treatment, and told it was just a matter of time until he would go to hospice care. In other words, there was no hope that he would recover.

Once I assumed responsibility for his care, I decided to conduct my own examination, because I needed to assess him for myself. He was no longer dependent on a ventilator, so he was breathing on his own by this time, but otherwise he was essentially non-responsive. As I approached his bed, I introduced myself to him, and as expected, there was no reply. I gently shook him and asked him to wake up, as I had been taught to do. I asked him to move his hands, his toes, to wiggle his fingers, or give me some sign of awareness. Although he did not respond to any of my commands, when I looked into his eyes, I saw... something. Call it a spark, a light, or simply a level of awareness, I could sense that a part of him was "there." Perhaps it was just wishful thinking.

Now this is where the story takes a strange turn. I remember that he was Egyptian, because my wife is also Egyptian, and I am able to speak a little bit of Arabic. In any case, his family was in the room as I was doing my examination. They had already come to terms with the fact that he was never going to wake up. Imagine their reaction when I told them, after having just taken over his care and reading his patient file for the first time, that I thought we were missing something. I began explaining to them that the brain sometimes does weird things after suffering a sudden shock, like a car accident, or other physical or emotional trauma. It's like it shifts into a protective mode, and when one part of the brain is injured, sometimes another takes over. I was really just talking to them about my fascination with the brain, and my hunch that something like this might be happening with Youssef.

I explained to them that sometimes after this kind of trauma the brain reverts back to its earliest memories and its earliest exposure to language. Knowing he was Egyptian, I asked Youssef's family if he spoke Arabic. They told me that he had moved here when he was two years old, and while his parents had spoken to him in Arabic as a young child, he had not spoken the language since then. I was told he was as American as anyone else and had only spoken English for the past twenty-five years. I listened to them, but inside, for some reason, I felt that I was on to something. Sensing their skepticism but ignoring it, I pressed on. I asked if they would try to say something to Youssef in Arabic, because up to that point we were all speaking English. The more I talked the more agitated his family became, until finally they were unable to contain their annoyance.

"Why are you giving us this false hope?" his sister demanded, as tears pooled in her eyes. "We already know he is gone, you don't need to do this," she continued.

I knew what I was asking was unconventional, but I had to follow through with this theory for my patient's sake. I told them they might be right, but we had nothing to lose by trying. Finally, his aunt began to slowly speak to him in Arabic. She said his name, then asked him to wake up, and told him she was there. Suddenly, Youssef's eyes opened, and he looked at her, then he began to look around the room. There was a collective gasp from everyone—including myself, no doubt, and then all eyes turned to look at me in shocked disbelief. Smiling, I encouraged Youssef's family to continue talking to him, and all six family members started speaking to him in Arabic all at once.

"Move your fingers," his aunt told him.

"Try wigging your toes!" his sister suggested.

"Can you blink to show you hear us?" asked his uncle.

Things didn't happen all at once for Youssef, but that day served as the catalyst for his recovery. Little by little, things started coming back to him. He began with little movements, and being able to follow simple instructions, and continued to improve from there. By the time my rotation was finished, and I signed over his care to another doctor, Youssef was able to speak and barely walk. I was pleased to see him doing so well.

A few months later I was working in my clinic, finishing up with a patient when a tall man in a baseball cap approached me from behind, and asked me my name. I turned to face him and as soon as I told him who I was, the man hugged me. I awkwardly asked him who he was, and with a big grin, he told me.

"My name is Youssef, and you saved my life," the man told me as tears ran down his cheeks.

I was speechless. I would never have recognized him as the man I had treated months ago. The man before me looked healthy and vibrant and was walking pretty well.

"I owe you," he said thanking me profusely and hugging me again.

The patient I had been with when Youssef walked in smiled at us both, thanked me for the consult, then exited the clinic. This gave me some time to catch up with my former patient. He told me how his recovery had been going and asked me how I had known what to do to help him. I told him that I believed the imprint we make in childhood has a special place in our brain. It's like those memories from childhood get preserved, and you just need a spark for them to come back to you. He was living proof that this sort of thing could happen.

Before Youssef left, he turned to me and asked if I would do one more thing for him. I looked at him questioningly, and he slowly removed his baseball cap.

He turned his head and said to me, "My head looks kind of funny. Can you fix it for me?"

You will recall me saying that surgeons would often not replace the portion of the skull they removed when the patient was not expected to survive? In Youssef's case, they had removed half of his skull, and had never put it back. When brain swelling goes down, it actually caves in a bit, so it did lend an unusual shape to his head. He had been walking around all this time missing half his skull! I agreed to help him, and with the help of my colleagues, we were able to create a 3D reconstruction of the part of the skull that was missing. I was the one who put his skull back in and closed his scalp up again.

Youssef looked great following the surgery. It was so hard to believe this was the same man everyone had given up on all those months ago. While he may have had some residual deficits as a result of his accident, he went on to live a relatively normal life.

The experience was humbling for me, and it taught me to always follow my gut and trust my instincts. That lesson has served me well ever since.

CHAPTER 3

Racing

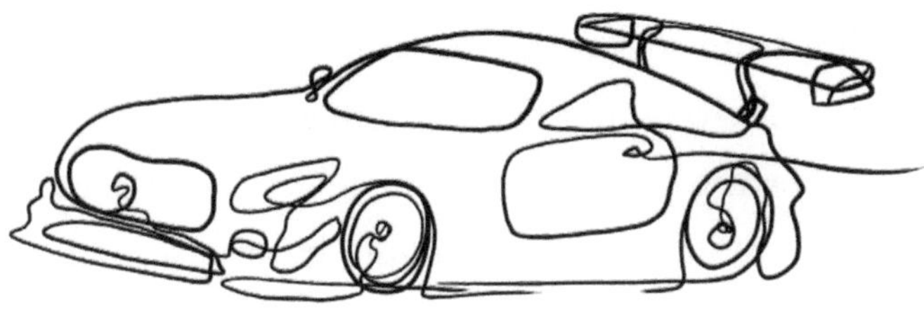

Being a doctor brings me face to face with people from all walks of life. From time to time, I meet celebrities and other famous people, although most of the time I don't know they are famous until someone else tells me. On more than one occasion, my kids have berated me when they learned I'd treated someone famous.

"Dad! Why didn't you get their autograph!" they'd demand.

One day a man came into my office complaining of a neck problem. I don't recall the man's name, so let's call him Joseph. He had been experiencing chronic neck pain, which had been getting worse and had started causing numbness and tingling down his arm. As it turns out, this man was a famous race car driver—although he was semi-retired when I met him. After the initial examination, I ordered an MRI and other tests to identify the source of his problem. Once I knew what was wrong, I recommended surgery. He agreed, and shortly after, I performed a neck fusion surgery on his spine. The surgery was a success but healing from it is a slow process because the bone fusion takes time to fully strengthen.

Following his surgery, I scheduled Joseph to come in regularly so I could monitor the progress of his recovery. Each time I met with him, I'd order x-rays to see how well the surgical area was healing and fusion was proceeding.

If there's one thing that stood out about Joseph it was his love of racing. He was a personable man and always pleasant to deal with, but he was as passionate about the sport of racing as I am about neuroscience. It was very difficult for him to sit on the sidelines and not race while his body recovered. I imagine I would feel the same way if I ever broke my hand and could not do surgery.

Joseph always came to his appointments with his wife, Jillian, who he'd been happily married to for over thirty years. Happily married or not, I could tell Joseph wasn't thrilled that his wife accompanied him to his appointments. During each visit Joseph would inquire how much longer it would be before he could get back to racing. His efforts to convince me to change my professional opinion didn't bother me at all. I would never be swayed by an argument that was not in the best interest of my patient. I never saw Joseph's cajoling as "nagging," as Jillian put it. I saw patients every day who were not feeling their best. I developed a tough skin very early on in my career and learned to take the negative things patients sometimes said with a grain of salt. Not that Joseph was one of these patients. Quite the opposite. He was never negative. But he had a big personality. I found him quite entertaining as a matter of fact—not that I would ever tell him that.

"So, it looks like things have healed up pretty nicely, haven't they doc?" Joseph said at his very first follow up appointment. I was about to answer when he added, "Looks like I'll be able to hit the track again, huh?"

"Joseph let the doctor speak," Jillian said, looking at him sternly when he opened his mouth to say something else.

"Things are looking good, but it's going to take time," I said, looking from him to his wife.

"Doc, you're killing me here. I feel fine," he said with what I'd come to recognize as his signature style of charming bravado.

"For goodness' sake Joe, listen with your ears not your mouth!" Jillian responded to save me from having to answer.

I explained what would be expected in terms of his recovery timeline and set up the next follow up appointment.

Over the next several visits, each time Joseph and Jillian walked into my office, before they'd even sat down, Joe would ask, "How soon till I can get back to racing?" I would do my assessment and tell him it was too soon. I guess you could say it became our routine.

A few months into his recovery, Joseph skipped the usual question about racing. Instead, he said, "I know, I know, you're going to say I can't race again yet." I noticed he had altered the pitch of his voice at the last part and smiled inwardly as I recognized his attempt to imitate my voice. "I have an ex— er, that is to say I have this show to do in a few weeks." He finished, then stopped and looked at me expectantly.

I had not yet figured out what this had to do with me, so I told him that was nice, and waited for him to continue.

Jillian elbowed him in the ribs and said, "Tell him what it really is."

Joseph looked pained, though whether from the elbow or his reticence to be forthcoming I wasn't sure. He said, "Okay, okay, it's not really a show. It's more like an exhibit—"

Again, Jillian elbowed him and said "He doesn't know what you're talking about. Tell him what it is!"

Joseph started inching away from his wife. "Okay, well it's a sort of a driving exhibition coming up next month, but really we're just supposed to be showing the cars," he said. "It's just a bunch of us older, retired drivers who are basically showing these cars around our track..." He had managed not to use the word "race" once.

With a snort, Jillian decided she'd been patient long enough. She looked at him with exasperation and said, "It's a race Joe! Tell him it's a race!" Now we were getting somewhere.

Joseph gave his wife an offended look, then clarified. "No, it's not a race, Jillian. It's an exhibition," he said. I noticed absently he was now out of range of his wife's elbow.

"How fast are you driving in this exhibition?" I asked him.

"Um, well we're probably going to average about 120 miles an hour." He answered.

"That kind of smells like a race to me," I said. "You're not ready to race again," I told him firmly.

The next visit, I had to choke back a laugh when he walked in. He was carrying a neck brace contraption, which I would soon be informed is called a HANS device (head and neck support device). Misreading my expression, Joseph said, "Don't say it doc. I know you'll say it's too soon. I just wanted you to see how safe these racing harnesses are."

It was an interesting learning experience for me because I'd never seen that type of contraption before. Joseph demonstrated how the brace was put on. It goes across the driver's shoulders and braces their neck and head to limit it from moving around. He was trying to make a strong case for why he could still race cars. He showed me the finer points of the harness, and answered my questions in great detail, simultaneously ignoring his wife's exaggerated eye rolls.

The great thing about all the time that had passed since his surgery is that he'd been steadily healing. Joseph's neck fusion had been getting stronger as the bone hardened. Each time he'd come in and made his arguments, I'd told him he was not ready, but I could see the progress he was making during each visit.

X-ray after x-ray proved the bone had been solidifying and he'd been getting stronger and stronger.

Now that it was almost time for his exhibition race, he was finally ready. His spine was fused and healed and I was able to give him the "green light" to proceed. I wish I had a photo of the look on his face when I finally told him it was time. He looked like a child in a candy store. He shook my hand rigorously, then pulled me in for a hug. I wondered if he was going to cry. Jillian beamed with happiness, and I could see the love she had for him reflected in her eyes. Joseph went on to do his race and said it went very well. He sent me pictures and a note of thanks for giving him the opportunity to do what he loved again. As if anticipating the unspoken question, he'd added, "Exhibitions don't have winners."

Below this was a flowery line of script, which I presumed was Jillian's handwriting. It read, "He means he came in third!"

CHAPTER 4

The Makeover

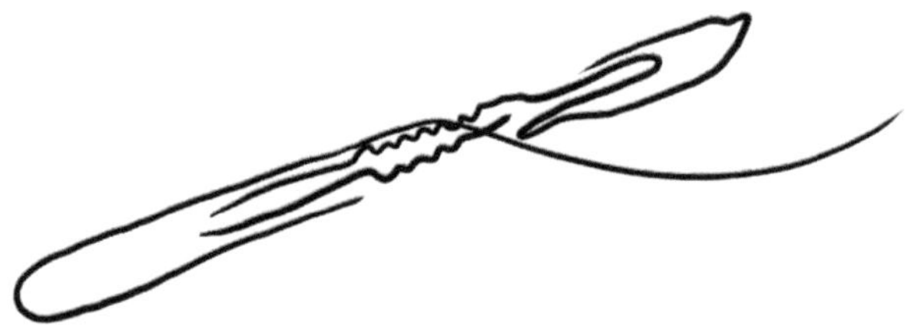

I was on rotation on the plastic surgery service when I was given a very strange assignment. Each day when I arrived at the hospital for my shift, I would be given the name of my first patient. For plastic surgery cases, a history is usually provided to explain the reason the patient was there. There might be any number of scenarios for why a patient would need plastic surgery; for example, they might have been in a car accident and suffered from some sort of disfigurement, or they may have had cancer surgery and needed some reconstructive surgery. On this particular morning, I was given the name of my patient as was the routine, and then I was told I was to go see the patient and prep them for surgery. I immediately knew this was going to be an unusual case. First off, the patient's name was listed as John Doe. The name John or Jane Doe is often given to a patient when we don't yet know the patient's identity, or in order to protect someone's identity. Another strange detail was that the floor where the patient was located was typically no longer in use. It had been closed for many months. Maybe I would be working on a celebrity today, I thought.

The elevator, it turned out, would not stop on the floor I selected, so I got off on the floor above and took the stairs down a flight. As I approached the floor, an unfriendly looking man in a dark suit stared at me from his position in front of the access door to the floor. He looked like the FBI agents you see on TV. As it turns out, he was an FBI agent, and he would not let me onto the floor until he had triple checked my ID, and then verified my purpose. When I was finally allowed to enter, it felt like I'd entered a scene out of a movie. There were police officers, FBI agents and a number of official-looking security people standing in the hallway at the entrance and exit points to the floor, as well as in front of the room where my patient was located. I was starting to think my patient was not the kind of celebrity I would invite to a dinner party.

My patient was in handcuffs and chains and was lying in bed when I entered the room. Another guard was standing behind him when I entered the room. He moved back a short distance when I approached. My patient was an older gentleman, who looked to be in his late sixties or early seventies. I could see why he wanted surgery—he had a lot of what we would call "historical disfigurement." His face was heavily scarred and had a lot of keloid and other types of oddly healed skin that were clearly the result of past injuries.

In contrast to his appearance, he was very mild mannered.

"Good morning doctor," he said politely.

"Good morning—sir," I responded.

"So, you're the miracle worker who's going to fix my face then?" he said.

"It looks that way," I answered, smiling. He was very pleasant to talk to.

"Can you make me look like Brad Pitt?" he joked as I consulted his sparsely populated patient chart.

"How about George Clooney?" he continued, clearly enjoying himself.

"I'll do my best," I answered with another smile, and then got on with the business of preparing him for surgery.

I wondered what this amiable old man had done to deserve such a robust security contingent...or how he got those scars for that matter. It is probably for the best that I didn't find out until after I'd completed his surgery.

I would eventually find out, through the hospital grape vine, that my patient was an accused serial killer. He had been scheduled for trial but his attorney had argued that it would be impossible for his client to receive a fair trial because of his severe facial disfigurement. He'd claimed that any jury who saw his client would judge him based on his appearance rather than the facts of the case. The attorney had won the argument and so his client had been granted the requested surgery. I agree that everyone deserves a fair trial, but I'd never heard of such great lengths being taken to assure someone that they'd receive one. The cost of his surgery alone was significant, to say nothing of the logistical coordination and expense.

We (meaning my medical team and I) would not allow guards within the operating room, but they remained just outside the doors and ensured he remained in chains before and immediately following the surgery. The surgery itself took about five hours, and it was a success by all accounts. I wasn't a magician, but I'd done a good job of repairing and improving his facial appearance.

I never found out whether he was convicted of the crimes he'd allegedly committed; I guess I just didn't want to know. That night I stayed up long after my kids and wife had gone to bed. I was thinking about what I had heard about my patient's alleged crimes. It was incongruous with the image he had presented to me that morning. He'd seemed so...well, nice. I thought about everything I'd heard about famous serial killers in the news, and how police and neighbors would always say the person had been very charming and could not believe the person was capable of such atrocities. Serial killers are good at deceiving people, and that's how they draw in their prey. I was glad he'd have no grudge against me... unless of course he'd been serious about the Brad Pitt thing, I thought, joking inwardly. I finally decided it was time to head up to bed. Before I did however, I double checked the locks on the front and back door and made sure the security alarm was armed.

CHAPTER 5

Theo's Nightmare

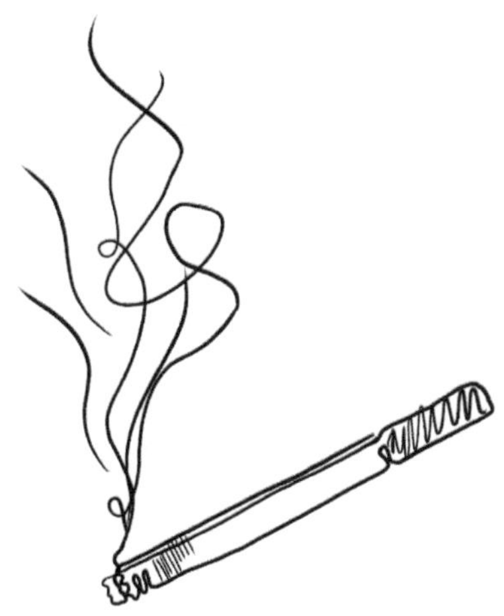

This story is a sad one, but it speaks to the strength of the human spirit. I was still an intern when Theo, a man in his mid-thirties was admitted in critical condition. Theo had fallen asleep while smoking, and his untended cigarette had started a fire in his bedroom. He was lucky to be alive. When he arrived at the hospital, he was suffering from third degree burns over most of his body, including his face and most of his torso, as well as his arms, legs, hands, and feet. The really awful thing about burn injuries is that in addition to the pain and damage they cause, the burn victim is prone to many potential complications. Among the most dangerous complications is the risk of infection because the skin is a natural protective layer and without it, there is no barrier from bacteria for example. Bleeding is another major concern. The primary goal for medical professionals in this type of case is always to prevent infection, prevent further damage to the affected areas and to try and close as much of the wounds as possible as soon as the patient is stable enough to do so.

Burns can be quite gruesome, depending on how much injury there is and the level of burn the patient has sustained. It can be shocking not only for the families of burn victims, but also for the hospital care staff, including doctors and nurses, to see patients who've been badly burned. This was the case for Theo.

Theo had been on the burn service for a couple of weeks when my rotation started and I took over responsibility for his care. Treatment for cases like Theo's include water-based therapy such as ultrasound mist to help clean the wounded tissue and stimulate the production of new tissue, infection prevention and pain management drugs, creams and ointments, dressings, and the administration and monitoring of internal hydration. Having survived the initial burn, Theo was now at the stage where we needed to start transplanting some of his skin from a "good" area of his body to a "bad" area. To do this, a surgeon will take several layers of skin thickness and graft it from an undamaged area, then move it to the patient's face, arms, or other priority areas. We began doing this little by little over the next several weeks, which allowed him to regain his strength at the same time.

Theo's hands had been severely affected by the fire and all the skin on his fingers had been burned. We needed to replace this skin, so we were doing small grafts onto his fingers. This type of graft is very delicate, and it requires the insertion of wires into the fingers so the patient cannot bend them. If the patient moves their fingers, it may destroy the grafts, causing the "good" skin to fall off. The wires look like needles and are very pointy and sharp, so we put little rubber stoppers at the ends, to make sure they don't accidentally injure the nurses and doctors. It takes about a week for split-thickness grafts to start to connect to the surrounding tissue, and a few weeks for the area the skin was grafted from to heal. The pins would stay in until the skin had fully attached and there was no longer risk of the new skin becoming detached.

There he was, very sick and in the intensive care unit, with burns all over his face and body. He was covered in white dressings, many of which were weeping red blood and other substances, and he had all these wires sticking out of the tips of his fingers. The image of him looking like this will haunt me for the rest of my days. I thought about how scary this must be for him and I felt a wave of sadness when I silently acknowledged how scary he looked to my colleagues, and even myself. He reminded me of Freddy Kruger from the 1980s movie *Nightmare on Elm Street.*

Up to that point Theo had not been able to wake up or talk yet, but the day came when it was time to remove his breathing tube. This was progress. A few days later, Theo began to wake up. One day soon after the tube had been removed, his nurse called me to say Theo had finally opened his eyes. When I arrived at his bedside, Theo was mumbling, but no one could understand what he was saying. I drew closer to him, mindful of the long, sharp wires still imbedded in his fingers, then leaned over to hear him better. I asked him to repeat what he was saying. I was curious to know what the first words might be for this poor man, in this sad situation. Perhaps it was something inspirational, or profound, or maybe he was simply asking about a family member. When I finally understood what he was saying, my heart felt like lead in my chest.

"Please kill me," he whispered, over and over.

I offered words that I hoped might comfort him, although I can no longer recall what they were. There are moments when doctors appreciate their own limitations. We were doing everything we could to help Theo recover, but some things went beyond physical care. If Theo were to recover, he had to *want* to live. I wondered how I would feel if it were me lying there in bed covered in bandages. I wasn't sure I'd feel any different than he was in that moment. Extensive psychiatric and psychological therapy would be part of his long-term treatment plan, and I made a note for his care team to monitor his mental state and notify me if anything changed. I could only hope that as Theo's body healed, his psychological outlook would also improve. Only time would tell.

Theo's family had not come see him yet because Theo refused to let them see him in his current state. He was afraid that the sight of him would be too disturbing. As Theo's body mended, he began to look less scary, and he allowed a few family members to begin to visit him regularly. This had a huge positive impact on his mental state. Theo, it turned out, had a wonderful sense of humor, and a very loving family.

Physical therapy is a critical part of a burn patient's rehabilitation. In the early stages of recovery, a physical therapist will focus on things like monitoring and adjusting the patient's body to prevent the contraction of tissue, which can happen as scar tissue develops over the damaged areas and can limit the patient's range of motion. They also monitor the elevation of the patient's limbs and position them so as to reduce swelling, do splinting, stretching, and focus on the prevention of pressure sores. As the patient gets better, the therapist will begin guiding the patient through limited exercises and movement to further encourage flexibility of the injured area. Theo's physical therapist worked to help him to rebuild his endurance, strength, and balance again. It was a very slow and painful process, but Theo rarely complained, even as tears streamed down his face and his arms and legs shook with the effort.

At first Theo was quiet and didn't interact much with staff and was very withdrawn. But as he regained his strength and was able to move around, his personality began to show. It helped that he had a psychologist as part of his health team. Mental health care was another integral part of Theo's rehabilitation. Eventually Theo started cracking the odd joke and laughing sometimes.

I was no longer Theo's primary doctor by the time Theo's bandages came off and he was able to walk. By then I had cycled through two other rotations, so it really was a slow road to recovery for him. I had remained interested in his case however and had been observing his progress from a distance. He would never look "normal" again, but it seemed his chances for a somewhat normal life had increased significantly.

It was a long road to recovery, but when Theo was finally released from the hospital, although still badly disfigured, he was mentally stronger and focused on getting back into the real world again. I can't say his was a fairy tale ending, but Theo taught me something important about the incredible resilience of the human spirit, and the critical part that mental attitude plays when it comes to any kind of recovery.

CHAPTER 6

Border Patrol

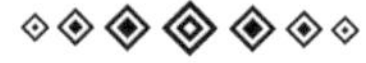

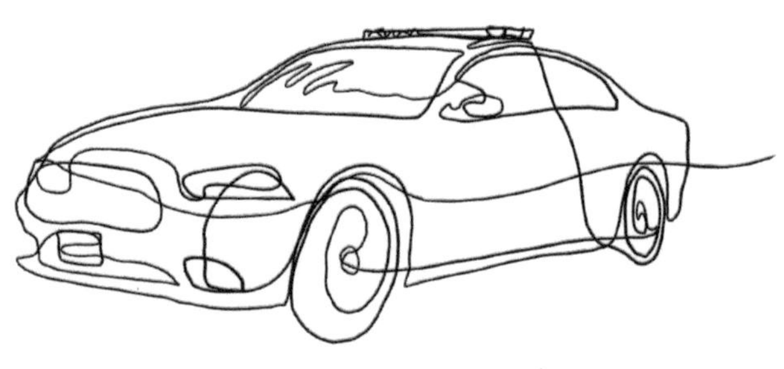

I did my residency in San Diego, which is very close to the Mexican border. Oftentimes ambulances and medical teams would come across people from Mexico who had been left at the border in need of medical attention. Family members would routinely drop off loved ones at the border because they knew they could get better medical care in the US. They would kiss their loved one goodbye, not knowing if they'd ever see them again. This in itself is sad, but it is downright tragic when the patients are children.

One day an ambulance brought in a young boy of about nine or ten years of age. He'd been found alone at the border, and he'd been picked up and brought in by ambulance. Sometimes in this type of situation the children would have family already living in the US, so they would be taken into that family member's custody once they were released from the hospital. Unaccompanied minors who didn't have a family member in the US would end up becoming a ward of the state.

The boy had told the ambulance attendants that his name was Mateo but had otherwise been very quiet and frightened. When he got to the hospital, I began talking to him to help him feel more at ease, and to obtain whatever information I could from him. Getting him to talk at all was difficult, but he did provide me with some basic information, which was useful for developing my initial assessment. I then ordered some tests to be done to help with his diagnosis and asked him if I could call somebody for him.

"I'd like to tell your mom and dad that you got here okay. Do you know their phone number?" I asked. Mateo just shook his head. Being a father of two children by then, my heart broke for the little guy. He looked so lost. A social worker would be assigned to look after him during his stay in the hospital unless or until a family member could be located and assume custody.

As it turned out, Mateo had a brain tumor. I realized his parents must have known or suspected this, and they had risked the possibility of never seeing him again for the chance to save his life. They would have known what they were doing was illegal but must have felt it was their only choice. Their sacrifice was one that no parent should ever have to make, but it is a sad reality for far too many.

Once I had confirmed Mateo's diagnosis, I again asked him if there was anyone I could call. He just looked at the floor and didn't answer. Thankfully, the next day, an older man showed up asking for Mateo. It was Mateo's uncle. He was a legal US resident and was able to speak on Mateo's behalf. Mateo's parents had arranged for him to care for Mateo while he was in the US. When I spoke to his uncle and shared the plans for Mateo's surgery, I kept thinking of how sad it was that his parents could not be there.

"I know his parents don't have the necessary paperwork to be here, but maybe there's something I can do to help." I said earnestly. I was not well versed in immigration law, but I knew that his parents could not be here unless they had legal documentation. I also understood better than most people what the risks were for Mateo undergoing this surgery. I kept replaying in my mind how anxious his parents must feel. I thought that as a doctor, I might be able to write a letter that Mateo's uncle could bring to immigration officials. I figured they might grant an exemption and allow his parents to come here if they understood Mateo's situation.

The uncle pulled me aside to a quiet corner of the hospital and sort of chuckled. He put a hand on my arm and gently said to me, "I appreciate you trying to help. But if we go through the legal route, it means a lot of paperwork and letters, and it will probably take a few weeks or a month before we get a response."

"Mateo can't wait that long," I said, finally understanding the complexity of his family's situation.

"Exactly," his uncle agreed. "If Mateo does not have that surgery now, he will die." He added. My face must have betrayed my feelings because he then winked. "Don't worry though," he said with a mischievous smile. "We have other means to reunite Mateo with his family.

"What do you mean?" I asked, curious.

"Let's just say there are unofficial ways to get them here." He answered, then added, "If they come here underground, they'll be here tomorrow."

I wonder what I must have looked like in that moment—whether I'd looked as shocked as I felt. The next morning, we performed Mateo's surgery.

Everything went well, and the tumor was benign. He suffered no damage from the surgery and was released from the hospital a few days later into his uncle's care.

It was not Mateo's condition or surgery that made this story stay with me. It was the fact that I had been trying to help Mateo and his family by the only means I knew how. Legalities and bureaucracy notwithstanding, at the end of the day I was hopeful that a little boy facing major surgery would soon be reunited with his family.

CHAPTER 7

A Second Opinion

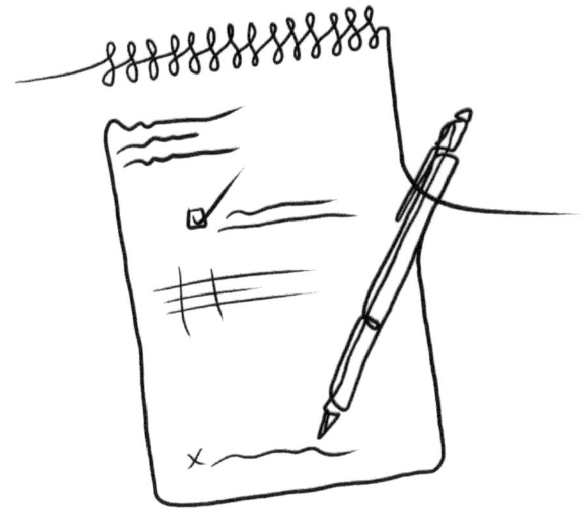

My least favorite part of this job is dealing with insurance companies and the bureaucracy around insurance authorizations. People who don't have a medical background should not be making decisions about the kind of medical treatment a patient is allowed to receive. Ethically we know it shouldn't be this way, but this is the sad reality of our healthcare system. As such, there are times when I have to fight for my patients. Navigating the bureaucracy and arguing to an insurance administrator with little to no understanding of medical science about the finer points of why a patient should not be denied coverage can be exhaustive and very frustrating. But sometimes patients need a champion, and I am not shy to advocate on their behalf when I feel it is appropriate and necessary.

Before I go any further, I want to explain the distinction between neurology and neurosurgery. Although there is a lot of overlap between the two, there are some key differences. A neurosurgeon is essentially a neurologist with additional surgical training. They are licenced to perform surgery. A neurologist can still diagnose and treat neurologic problems, but they are not surgeons. I point this out because it will help you to better understand the issues the patient and myself faced in this next story.

A patient named Brian came to me with complaints about his neck, arm, and leg. When multiple parts of the body are involved, it's important to take a step back and ascertain where the problem is stemming from. You have to figure out if it is a number of isolated problems or if it is all the result of one underlying issue. In this patient's case, I had to rule out a number of possibilities. For example, could the numbness and tingling be the result of diabetic neuropathy? Or could it be a central nervous system issue stemming from the brain or spinal cord that was causing problems for the whole body? I would need to do a thorough examination and see Brian's patient and family history to know more.

After examining Brian, I had a suspicion about what the problem might be, but I needed to know more before I could make a diagnosis. I ordered an MRI to help me figure things out. I also ordered an electromyography (EMG) test. An EMG is a nerve test, where a neurologist will insert little needles into the patient to test nerve function. Doing this test would help me narrow down the diagnosis even further. When Brian came back to me, having completed these tests, I read the results of the MRI first, but could not see anything unusual. This was curious. I asked myself how he could have all these significant complaints if I couldn't see a problem on his MRI? There had to be something else going on, I thought. And so, I turned to the results of the EMG.

The neurologist who had performed the nerve test was insurance authorized, and his findings said that it was some kind of lumbar spine issue. This did not make sense to me. My intuition told me there was something more serious going on with this patient. And the MRI of Brian's brain and spine did not support the neurologist's findings. I had to consider that the neurologist was mistaken. There was another, very skilled neurologist that I knew, and I decided Brian should have another EMG done with him. Finding a more experienced doctor to do the test was the easy part. Getting insurance authorization for it would prove to be a great deal more challenging.

I cannot count how many hours I spent explaining and reexplaining why I needed to repeat Brian's nerve test. Each time I wrote to or called the insurance company, I'd be told that the neurologist who had conducted the test was experienced. And each time I would write back or tell the dispassionate voice on the other end of the call that Brian needed a more experienced neurologist to conduct the test because I suspected there was something else wrong. The insurance company ignored my arguments and kept refusing my repeated request. The mandate of insurance companies is incongruous with that of medical professionals. They were concerned about their bottom line, whereas I had my patient's best interest at heart. Time and again, they'd tell me I already had a nerve test done for him and they'd decline my request. They'd tell me if I disagreed with their decision I would have to appeal. And so, I'd appeal. I felt like we were going in circles, and I was beginning to lose hope.

The last call I made, I decided to be completely candid in my response. I was speaking to someone much higher up on the food chain by this point. I told them, "All surgeons are not equal. Not all neurologists are equal. And not all tests are equal. Something else is going on with this patient and I don't trust the results of the EMG that was done."

As luck—and my dwindling patience—would have it, the test was finally approved.

The neurologist the insurance company had approved was far less experienced than the one I had recommended. The new neurologist did the test and sent me the report, but also urgently called me on the phone to share the results. His diagnosis confirmed my suspicion. Brian had a devastating disease called Amyotrophic Lateral Sclerosis (ALS).

ALS is also known as Lou Gehrig's disease, named after a famous New York Yankee's baseball player who was diagnosed with it in the late 1930s. It is a neurodegenerative condition, which affects the central nervous system. With ALS a patient loses almost complete neurologic function; the nervous system deteriorates very quickly and they usually die. There is no surgery for it, but there are medications that can help with some of the symptoms, and physical therapy may also help as well.

It's a very important diagnosis to make, because if the disease process is missed and/or the wrong diagnosis is suspected, it might mean the patient gets surgery for something they didn't need—a surgery that won't help them. It's critical to identify the correct diagnosis as soon as possible because the patient and their family will have no idea what is going on, and this can lead to more and more problems. Sometimes, by the time the disease is diagnosed, patients have very little time left. Although the disease is relatively rare, it is so devastating it should never be missed, but it happens. Patients may pass away without ever discovering what was wrong with them, potentially having wasted whatever precious time they might have had left.

I was sad that I was right. I was also very upset with the insurance company, not to mention the original neurologist who had been trying to talk Brian into having surgery when so clearly it would not have helped. The time between when Brian first noticed symptoms and when he received his diagnosis took about six months. About three of those months were wasted arguing with the insurance company about their decision to deny the second nerve test. When somebody has a terminal diagnosis, every day counts. That is what made the ordeal so extremely frustrating to me.

Brian came to see me again a few months after he had come to terms with his diagnosis. I was pleased to see him still up and about. We chatted for a few minutes and then he said, "I want to thank you for helping me. No other doctor knew what it was, and they kept sending me down rabbit holes that were just wasting time."

He told me that finally having a diagnosis, and knowing the name of the disease he had, had enabled him to get the treatment and therapy he needed.

I wish I could say Brian had a miraculous recovery, but this was not the case. Brian died about two years later, at home, surrounded by his family. That thought, at least, brought me comfort that he was with his family and he didn't undergo an unnecessary surgery.

I learned a lot about the power of persistence from my experience arguing with the insurance company on Brian's behalf. It would have been so easy to give up the first time the insurance company said no. Even easier the second, third and fourth time. It can feel daunting, even to a seasoned medical doctor. But I learned the value of not giving up; it's a lesson I hope others will be inspired by as well.

CHAPTER 8

Cultural Sensitivity

◇◈◆◈◆◈◇

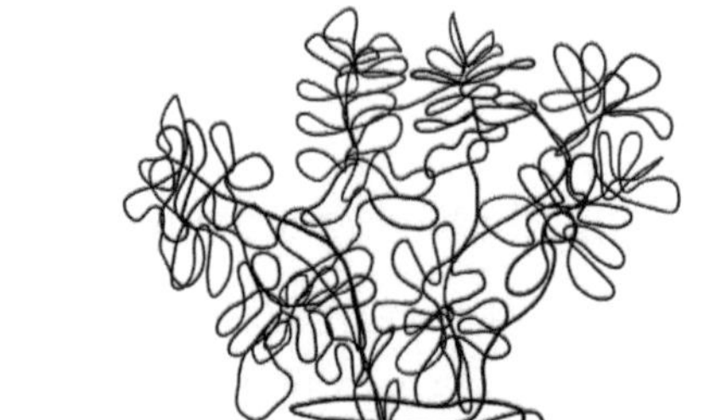

You will notice many of the stories I have included in this book are from the days when I was still an intern. As you may have guessed, this is because in those days I was rotating through the many different service areas of the hospital and therefore seeing patients coming in with a wide variety of conditions and ailments.

This next story is about Mrs. Wang, a petite, eighty-two-year-old Chinese woman who lived with her children and grandchildren. In Chinese culture it is common to see multiple generations of a family living in the same household. Older people are greatly respected for their wisdom, and because of this they remain an integral part of their families and society. Traditionally, elderly people in China are consulted before any major decisions are made. It is a lovely aspect of their culture, showing honor and respect.

When Mrs. Wang came in for her appointment, she was accompanied by her two granddaughters, Mei, and Liu. Mrs. Wang did not speak English, so she needed them to translate our conversation. Mei told me her grandmother was here to have a lump on her breast examined. Even though Mrs. Wang was wearing an oversized sweater, I could easily see a large, lumpish protrusion on her chest. When Mrs. Wang removed her sweater and undershirt for me to do an examination, I was shocked. The skin around the lump on her left breast had an orange hue and was very lumpy. There is a French term for this condition, called "peau d'orange," which literally means orange peel. It is a fitting term because the skin looks like the rind of an orange. I was not shocked at the appearance of the area, having seen this condition before; it was the size of the tumor that surprised me. It was huge. It had gotten so big that it looked like it was rolling out of her skin. I could not believe this had gone unnoticed and undiagnosed before now.

"When did you first notice this condition, Mrs. Wang?" I asked. Mrs. Wang started to reach for her clothing as Mei translated my question. She didn't answer or look at me.

"My grandmother did not tell us." Liu responded. "We only noticed it last week. When we asked, she said it was nothing," she continued.

"Our grandmother hid it from us. She wore baggy shirts and sweaters," Mei added.

Mrs. Wang admitted she had hidden her condition from her family because she did not want to be a burden on them. She had not wanted to worry them and did not want to cause them to go to any trouble on her behalf. I could see that just being at the hospital was difficult for her.

I ordered some tests, which confirmed what I had suspected. Mrs. Wang had a rare and aggressive form of breast cancer. If caught early, a patient's chances of survival from this type of cancer is reasonable. But in Mrs. Wang's case, treatment would only extend the limited amount of time she had left. With a heavy heart, I met with Mrs. Wang and her granddaughters again to give them the news in person. After sharing the test results with Mei and Liu, I waited for them to translate the information for Mrs. Wang. Although they did say something to their grandmother, the woman did not react as I expected. Rather than looking concerned, she nodded at me and smiled, then reached for her coat as if the appointment was over.

"Does she understand what we are telling her?" I asked, concerned.

"Yes," responded Mei, not looking at me.

It is important to note here that cultural background can affect how a person interacts with their doctor. Some cultures are more reserved than others, and there are many factors that come into play. I have given bad news to some people who immediately would break down crying. Other times, they've expressed anger, disbelief, or shock. Something about Mrs. Wang's behavior in that moment seemed off. Having just been given a diagnosis of having terminal cancer because the studies had shown that it had metastasized or spread extensively, I would have expected some sort of reaction. Something told me her granddaughters were not being truthful with me.

"Are you sure your grandmother understands the gravity of her situation?" I asked. As a doctor, it is my responsibility to provide patients with their diagnosis and treatment options. If the patient was not informed of their condition or choices, their right to choose was being denied.

Mei and Liu looked at each other then back at me.

"Can you give us a few minutes?" Liu asked me.

I nodded, then stood up and left the office, closing the door behind me. It was possible they wanted to break the news to their grandmother in private. I would allow them as much time as they needed.

When I returned to the office, about ten minutes later, all three women looked remarkably composed. The tissue box on my desk had not been disturbed and there were no red-rimmed eyes, tears, or sniffling. These women are stronger than I would be in their shoes, I thought to myself.

"Are we ready to discuss treatment options?" I gently asked the women.

"The thing is—" Mei began.

"The thing you need to understand," Liu interrupted, giving her sister a quick look of apology for cutting her off, then continuing. "My grandmother hid her condition from us because she does not want to be a burden. It was very difficult to even get her to come here today. She was very worried that we would be taking time off work to take her to appointments."

I looked at Mrs. Wang, who smiled and nodded at me again. She had no idea what we were talking about.

"She has told us many times she will not be a burden. She will never accept treatment. There is no question in our minds about this. I have already talked to my family and we all agree it is better not to tell her that anything is wrong," Mei continued.

Several concerns and possible responses came to my mind all at once, but I was experienced enough to really listen to what they were saying, and not to cut them off.

"Older people in my culture do not fear death. They accept it as a natural part of life," said Liu.

"Yes. And if we do not tell my grandmother, she will accept what is happening to her as a normal part of old age." Mei agreed.

"My parents also think this is how she would want it. She will not accept any treatment you offer and this way she can be happy until she dies." Liu finished.

I could see the women cared for their grandmother and their heart was in the right place. I could even understand their perspective on a personal level. Mrs. Wang was going to die either way, and this way she could live out her remaining days without the side effects of treatment or the shadow of imminent death hanging over her. But I was obligated to ensure that as my patient, Mrs. Wang understood her situation and was allowed to make that decision herself. I communicated as much to Mei and Liu.

The women looked at each other for a long moment, then turned their attention back to me.

"We will tell her now," Liu said gravely. Mei nodded in agreement.

Mrs. Wang was inspecting the visibly dehydrated jade plant on the edge of my desk, having lost interest in our conversation.

The women spoke to their grandmother, and I watched as Mrs. Wang's face registered first shock and then sadness. She bowed her head. I felt like the biggest jerk in the world at that moment.

"Did you tell her about her treatment options?" I asked.

Mrs. Wang looked up at my face when I spoke, and then at Liu for the translation. Liu spoke for a while and Mrs. Wang shook her head and said something sharply to her granddaughter.

"She only wants to go home." Liu said sadly.

I felt terrible for Mrs. Wang and her family and thought about them several times after that last appointment. Driving home that night, I had an urge to call my own grandmother and tell her I loved her. I did not choose this career so I could make old ladies cry, but sometimes it was inescapable.

Years later, I was at a dinner party with my wife, and I had just finished telling the story of Mrs. Wang (names and details withheld out of respect for patient privacy of course). It was an interesting case with cultural and ethical considerations, and I suppose I was curious to know how others might have reacted in those circumstances. The discussion was animated, but a single offhanded joke made me realize my guilt about insisting that Mrs. Wang be told of her condition may have been misplaced.

"They probably made up something that would get a reaction because you were watching. I bet they never told their grandmother at all," joked my wife's friend Tina.

I suddenly remembered the last thing the women had said to me when they exited the office that day.

"My grandmother says your jade plant needs water," Mei had said and smiled just before she closed the door.

Would a woman who had just found out she was dying be thinking about her doctor's plants? I wondered. I realized I would never know.

CHAPTER 9

The First Code

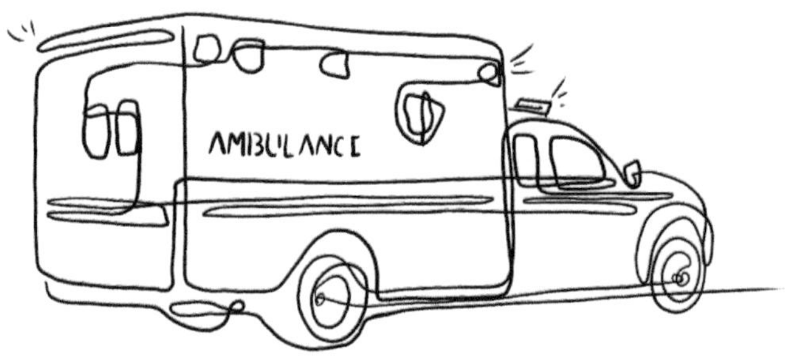

Have you ever been in a hospital and heard a "code blue," or code of some other color called over the public address (PA) system? Maybe you noticed hospital staff rushing somewhere after hearing one of these announcements. Did you wonder where they were going? For the benefit of anyone who has ever wondered, a hospital emergency is called a code. There are different types of codes to describe the kind of emergency that is occurring. If someone's heart stops, for example, a "code blue" would be called. There are code teams whose job it is to respond to these codes, and each member of the team has a specific task that they are responsible for. One person will be responsible for the defibrillator, another will bring the crash cart (a mobile unit that contains the materials and drugs needed to respond to a code), and so on.

The very first code I was involved with happened while I was still a medical student. I was about twenty-four-years-old at the time, and since I hadn't finished medical school and was not a doctor yet, I was only there to observe. Unfortunately for me, the first code I ever observed was also the first death I had ever witnessed.

This particular code occurred in the emergency room, so I ran there when I heard the call over the hospital's PA system. The scene that greeted me when I entered the ER looked like something out of the movies. Picture the worst scene in any hospital drama you've ever watched, and that's exactly what it looked like. It was probably the worst scene I have ever witnessed, not just because of all the drama, but because it was all happening in real time, right in front of me. The emotional aspect of this kind of situation is something you cannot fully appreciate unless you are there.

There were about twelve people huddled around a bed, doing different things. Given that I was only a medical student at that point, I did not yet understand all the different things that were going on, and there was a lot happening at once. The patient was a young lady who was visibly pregnant, and whose heart had stopped. The team around her was going through a sequence of procedures to try and save her life. They were giving her medications, shocking her heart, delivering chest compressions, monitoring her vital signs, and a number of other things all while calling out what they were doing, and talking to each other to try and figure out what was going on with her.

They were concerned about a number of things. For instance, it is unusual for someone so young to go into cardiac arrest. They were looking for clues to explain why this might have happened. The second concern was the fact that she appeared to be full term in her pregnancy. They needed to ascertain whether the baby was okay. Thirdly, there was the concern that they did not have her medical history. It is always a problem when someone comes into the emergency room for help and you don't know anything about them. Sometimes the only information medical staff are given is that the patient was discovered unconscious somewhere; they might not have identification with them, and the person who brought them in might not know anything about them or what happened.

In those cases, staff would work to track down their identification so they could contact the family, in hopes of ascertaining helpful information.

While all this was going on, I continued watching the doctors and nurses talking to each other while they worked. The energy in the room was palpable. They were becoming increasingly concerned that they had not yet been able to get her heart started. It was now becoming more of a concern that the baby might be in distress. Medical teams often have to make decisions very quickly, running through a number of steps to put the pieces of information they have together as best they can.

An obstetrics team was brought in to focus on the medical needs of the baby. They determined that an emergency caesarean section (C section) was required. If the mother's heart was not pumping, it meant the baby was getting no blood circulation either. The first team continued to focus on the upper half of the woman, pumping her heart, and administering the drugs and chest compressions. The second team performed the C section and took the baby out. A third team, also from obstetrics, came onto the scene and began working on the tiny baby that the second team had delivered. The baby was blue when it came out and was not breathing. As the third team labored to resuscitate the child, the second team began sewing up the mother's uterus, having successfully completed the C section. To witness everything at once was overwhelming for me. When I would ask questions about what had happened, nobody seemed to know.

Eventually, the first team reached the point where it was necessary to give up their attempts at resuscitation. In spite of their heroic efforts, they'd been unable to restart the mother's heart. There is a certain amount of time allocated for this kind of thing, and if there is no response and nothing is happening by then, the protocol requires that they "call the code." I heard a doctor say there was nothing more they can do for the mother, and that they had to pronounce her dead. Several people, including people on the code team who had a lot of experience with this sort of thing, broke down crying. Never mistake clinical disassociation for lack of caring. Medical staff care deeply about the welfare of their patients. This kind of situation is emotional for everyone, especially when someone very young dies. Although I had not been part of the woman's rescue team, I too could not stop the tears, as it hit me that someone had just died, right there in front of me.

I had to now focus my attention on the team working on the baby. The newborn child was still blue and the color was not fading in spite of the team's valiant efforts. They finally had to call the baby's death as well. I'd been so excited to see my first call. But this was not at all what I had expected. I couldn't stop the tears this time, but then, I was in good company. We all felt this tragedy. My very first call had been a double code, and both patients had died. It was by all counts a terrible experience.

My inquisitive mind wondered what had just happened? Young healthy people don't have hearts that just stop for no reason. I kept replaying what had happened in my mind, searching for clues. I resolved to investigate the case further. Nobody really knew what had happened. I was informed there would be an autopsy of the mother's body, and that it might shed some light on things.

The autopsy revealed that the mother had a rare tumor called a pheochromocytoma. This type of tumor secretes certain hormones into the body. Normally, we have a normal level of these particular hormones, which regulate our heart rate, our circulation, some of our sex hormones and other things that keep our bodies in balance. This particular tumor secretes extra amounts of these hormones, which causes heart palpitations, can boost your blood pressure, and other negative symptoms. It emits sudden flushes of these drugs (hormones) into the bloodstream, and although they are drugs that are natural to the human body, it's too much up or too much down. It's like having a thermostat that keeps getting cranked all the way up and then cranked all the way down; your body is constantly out of balance, unable to regulate itself.

I went back to take a look at the mother's obstetric and gynecologic chart and saw that she had been seeing a doctor throughout her pregnancy. When I read through her chart, it showed that at every appointment, she had complained about something, from hot flashes to a racing heart, to headaches and backaches. The trouble is, as many women who have gone through pregnancy will say, these symptoms are very common. Her doctor did not feel that there was anything abnormal happening. The other tragedy about this case was that the tumor, which was located in her abdominal area, was really quite large. It was the size of a large grapefruit, and had she not been pregnant it would have been quite noticeable, and therefore very easy to detect. Because she'd been so far along in her pregnancy, nobody bothered feeling around; her doctor had been focused on the baby. It was a horrible twist of events.

We would later learn that the woman's family had called 911 after she had passed out at home. It had never happened to her before, so naturally they'd been very alarmed. They had followed the ambulance to the hospital and had been waiting for an update on her condition. I watched as the doctor in the hallway broke the news to the woman's husband and other family members. Their immediate reaction was shock and disbelief, and then everyone collapsed in grief. I turned away, telling myself it was out of respect for their privacy and had nothing to do with the tears that had begun to well up in my eyes once again.

When things like this happen in the hospital, counseling is usually offered, sessions will be arranged so that staff can talk about the code. Also there are case and "M&M" conferences. "M&M" stands for morbidity and mortality. In these conferences, we discuss outcomes where there are complications or death. Everyone gathers in an auditorium or meeting room, and the case is presented. Doctors and nurses have the opportunity to talk about what happened and what they learned from it. It's an open presentation and discussion. People always want to know what they could have done differently. These sessions are helpful because they allow staff to learn from the experiences of others—both the mistakes and the successes as well.

I continued looking through her charts and realized there were many different pieces to her story. She had this tumor that had gone undetected because she was pregnant. Why was that? I wondered. She'd complained of so many things, but everyone assumed the symptoms were the normal side-effects of pregnancy. Because of this, they never did a thorough workup on her to rule out other causes, such as this one, which happened to be really rare. Her doctor did what he thought was right, and what would have been best for 99 percent of pregnant women. But he did not do certain extra tests.

This brings up the healthcare debate about how much testing should be done on someone. What happened to this woman very rarely occurs, but the fact is, once in a while it does happen. So, the question is, should you use limited resources and routinely test everyone who comes in? On the one hand, if you lose one or two people this way, you will think you should have done this test and more.

There are a couple of things I took away from the experience. The first was about the importance of teamwork. When you witness a code, you see a lot of people working together in a coordinated effort to save someone. Everyone has a job to do and they all do it. In these situations, each member of the team relies on their teammates to do their part to optimize the chances of a positive outcome and ultimately to be able to save lives.

Another important takeaway for me was that I should always do my best. Sometimes things might be missed, such as what happened in this woman's case, but always, with anything in life, it is important to keep doing your best. As a physician this is critical. If you work in a factory and you're assembling a mobile phone when you miss something, it may get sold and then malfunction, but that does not mean the difference between life and death. In medical practice there is a very small margin for error. If you miss something or make a mistake, especially in surgery, it could have dire consequences. This experience reminds me to be as conscientious, careful and detail oriented as I can with everybody, and to always do my best.

The final takeaway for me is one that I have grown to appreciate even more over the years. It's the importance of being able to talk to someone about your feelings and experiences. Holding everything in can negatively affect your ability to do your job, to say nothing of the effects it can have on your personal life. I am fortunate that I have always been able to talk to my wife about these things. Having her support, love, and compassion has been tremendously helpful not only for sad times, but also the exciting times as well.

CHAPTER 10

Grabbing Life By The Horns

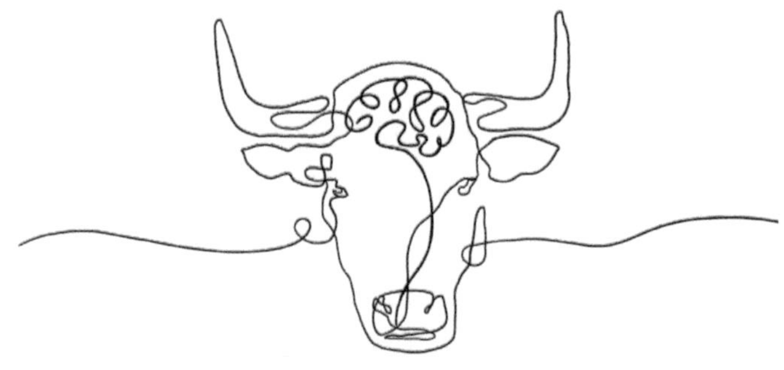

As a neurosurgeon, patients know that I commonly operate on the brain, the skull, and the spine. On the day this story took place, a patient with a very unique outward appearance walked into my clinic. He had an unusual hairstyle and clothing, and sported earspools, which I've learned are what you call those cylindrical earrings that make big holes in a person's earlobes. He also had lots of tattoos and piercings.

This patient did not have any neck pain or back pain. He did not have headaches. In fact, he had no neurologic complaints at all. I asked myself what he could possibly want from me? I politely asked him why he thought he needed the services of a neurosurgeon.

He told me, "I'm into body art and body modification, and I've been going to this guy who does all these piercings and things, but I'm ready to take things to the next level."

I realized he was waiting for me to say something. "Go on," I suggested, still at loss as to what he thought my role in all this would be.

"I've decided I want to have horns inserted into my skull," he said, then paused again, waiting for my response.

"You want horns inserted into your skull?" I repeated slowly.

"Yeah, there are tattoo parlours and piercing parlours that do that kind of thing now," he said, becoming animated. "They literally screw the horns into the skull," he added.

I digested this information, doing my best to keep my face neutral. I had heard of such things. Strangely, subdermal implants seem to be a growing trend for those seeking to add an element of shock value to their look. Apparently tattoos and piercings are not edgy enough for some people anymore. It is possible to implant the horns superficially into the skull so there would be little risk to the brain if done right. For this type of surgery a small incision would be made at the desired location, and then a dermal separator would be used to create space for the implant. The implant would be inserted and then the incision would be closed with sutures. It would not be a complicated surgery. It was his right to do what he wanted to his body, and it was not for me to judge. But as far as I was concerned this had nothing to do with me.

I told him, "That's your decision, but I don't do those kinds of things."

He said, "Okay, yeah, yeah I know. But because you're a neurosurgeon, and you work on skulls all the time, you're the safest person to put the horns on me."

I was impressed by his argument to have the surgery done in a sterile environment by a medical doctor but it was a hard no for me. "Sorry, I didn't go to medical school to put horns on people's heads. My focus is on saving people's lives," I said firmly. I wondered absently if this was perhaps a prank.

He tried to change my mind but he was wasting his breath. I was respectful and courteous, and it was an amicable appointment. He was disappointed and told me he would keep looking for a doctor to do it. I wished him good luck. I can't say whether or not he found another surgeon to do the procedure, or if he went back to his tattoo or piercing parlour. Whatever his decision, I hope he was safe and satisfied with the results. For me, I'll just pray that my children never come home with horns on their heads.

CHAPTER 11

Making The Diagnosis

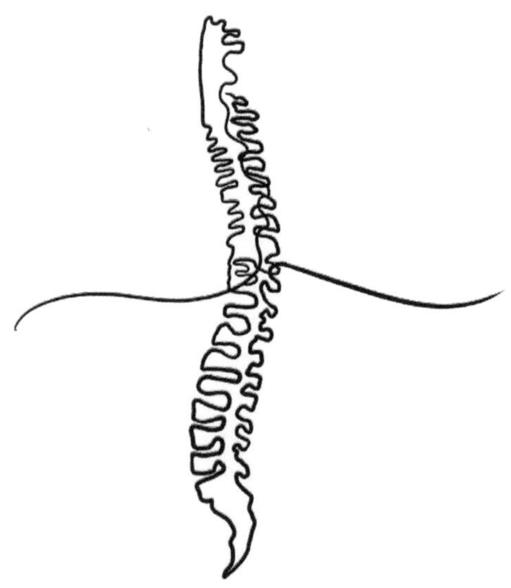

Sometimes patients come to me requesting a second opinion about a diagnosis they have received from another doctor. This was the case in my next story about a sixty-one-year-old woman named Nell, who came to me several years ago. Nell had been to see another surgeon who had recommended lower back surgery. She told me she'd sought me out because I had a good reputation, and she wanted someone to confirm whether the surgery was her best option.

As was the routine, I got her history, and did a physical examination of her. She told me that yes, her back and her legs hurt, then added that she also had some bowel and bladder complaints, and some issues in her lower chest area as well. During the examination, I began testing her strength as she walked, and going through a number of other tests that we do. It was clear she had a lower back issue, but my concern after completing the exam, was that there seemed to be something else going on. Usually when someone has a problem with their spine, the issues start from that point and travel downward. For example, if you have a problem in your lower lumbar spine, let's say around your hip area, then you would have pain around that area and down your legs. The issue usually did not typically radiate upwards. To me, this meant I would have to re-evaluate what was going on.

For those who may not know this, there are several sections to the spine. The chest level area of the spine is called the thoracic spine. Above that you have the cervical spine, which is the neck area. The lumbar spine is in the lower back, and this is the area where most people have problems. It is much less common to have problems in the thoracic spine. If a patient goes to a doctor complaining of back and leg pain, most doctors will order a lumbar spine MRI. If the MRI comes back confirming there are problems in the lumbar region of the spine, they will tell the patient there was a problem and may suggest surgery for that area, or else another remedy targeting that area. Unless the doctor is very thorough, they might not realize there is something else going on.

Based on Nell's history and exam, I was suspicious there may be an issue in the cervical or the thoracic area, so I ordered an MRI for each of those areas. Nell was a little annoyed with me. "Why do you want to do more MRIs?" she asked. "The other surgeon already did one of the lumbar spine and told me we have to do surgery."

I explained that it didn't make sense for her to have these upper body complaints as well as the bowel and bladder incontinence problems. I told her that her particular lumbar issue shouldn't cause such severe problems. She finally agreed to get the MRIs, but to be honest I didn't really expect to find anything new on them. I ordered them because I wanted to be sure I had ruled out every other possibility, and I make it a practice to be thorough. I was surprised when the MRIs came back and revealed she had a tumor in her thoracic spine. It was quite large actually, and when I saw it, all of the issues she told me she'd been experiencing made sense. Clearly, they were all related to the tumor, and it was not a lumbar spine issue at all.

She was shocked when I gave her the news, but also very grateful. "My god, if you or the other surgeon had done the lumbar surgery, you would have missed the thoracic tumor. It would have kept getting bigger and I would have continued to have problems," she said. She then gave me a hug and thanked me.

I explained the surgery to her so she would know what to expect, and then I answered her questions. I told her that there are many different types of tumors, and that I would not know what type hers was until I took it out. I'd have some idea of what sort of tumor we were dealing with when I saw it, but it would need to be sent to a pathologist for analysis before we could confirm anything. The pathologist would determine whether or not it was cancer and could tell us other details about the type of tumor it was. The most important thing for me would be to try and remove the whole tumor. Sometimes it's impossible to do so, for example if the tumor is attached to a part of the spinal cord or nerves. If I could remove it all, it would decrease the likelihood of the tumor ever growing back. Nell understood and was eager to move forward with the surgery. She told me she was ready to have her life back.

The surgery was a complete success and Nell did very well. I was pleased to have been able to get the entire tumor out. On top of this, the pathologist's report came back with good news—the tumor was benign. Nell did not have cancer, so she did not need any further treatment. I would still have her return to me every six months for follow up, to make sure the tumor never returned. It has been several years now, and there has still been no reoccurrence. Although completely unnecessary, Nell insisted on bringing me a batch of cookies after she'd recovered. (Sometimes there are perks to my job!)

If you are not satisfied with a diagnosis, you have the right to seek a second medical opinion. Nell's story might have had a different outcome if she had not done so. She also might not have had such a positive outcome if I had not been so thorough. My gut had told me I needed to puzzle things out and figure out why things didn't make sense. For me, this story underscores the need to investigate further if something doesn't fit, and to not be satisfied with the easy answer if the evidence does not completely support it.

Being reminded of this myself is one thing but telling a fellow surgeon that they missed something is another matter entirely. I knew it was a delicate matter, but I felt it was my duty to let the other surgeon know what had happened. In this instance, as luck would have it, the hospital where I worked happened to be holding a case conference on a related issue that I knew the other surgeon would be attending. The case conference was an opportunity to go over lessons learned, and I decided to present Nell's case to the attendees. It allowed me to highlight the need for more comprehensive workup and an accurate diagnosis without putting the surgeon on the spot. In the end, we are all human, but we can all learn from our mistakes.

CHAPTER 12

Doing The Right Thing

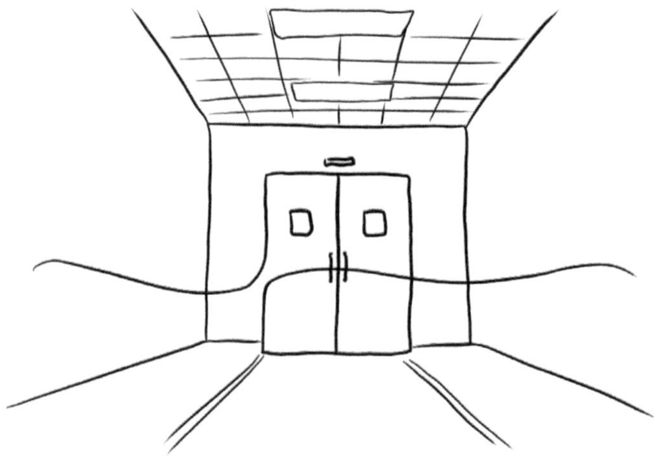

In many hospitals there is an area known as the trauma bay. It's where people who have undergone some sort of physical trauma are brought by the ambulance crew. This area may have all the equipment needed to do emergency surgery if it's required. Sometimes when people are brought in there is no time to run tests or do further diagnostics before operating. There may not be time to send a patient down for an MRI, for fear they might not make it. They could literally be dying in front of you. In the heat of the moment, especially in those first few moments after the patient is first brought in, you have precious little time to make big decisions.

I was an intern when this next story happened. I was doing a rotation on the trauma service when a patient was brought in following a car accident. He had sustained a lot of injuries all over his body.

The head trauma surgeon was there—he was a very tall, daunting, and aggressive figure with a very loud voice. He was directing staff about what to do, telling people to check the patient's extremities, listen to his heart, check his breathing, and so forth. He was giving orders the same way you would see it done when there is a code. It was very exciting for me to see how well orchestrated everything was.

While the surgeon was doing this, a systematic evaluation, known as a workup, was also being done. In a workup, there is what is called a primary and secondary survey. The primary survey focuses on the most important things, including the airway and circulation, to determine whether the patient is breathing, and circulation, to see if the patient's heart is pumping. It checks the most critical things required for body function. The secondary survey is the second level of evaluation. It is not as critical but still important. For example you would check the patient's arms and legs for broken bones and lacerations, and you would check to see whether they were bleeding out anywhere. As people were running through the surveys, they were announcing what they'd found and what they were doing about it as they addressed whatever issue they had found.

One of the things that you need to be concerned with in the trauma service is whether a patient has sustained any internal injuries. For example, if something has been torn in the bowel or colon, the patient could bleed out and develop an infection, and any number of things can happen in the belly. As the nurses and doctors were conducting the secondary survey and examining the patient's belly, they could not decide whether or not there'd been internal injury. Sometimes you can smell if there has been a bowel or colon injury. In this patient's case, the daunting and aggressive trauma surgeon started sniffing the air and determined that he could smell bowel. This indicated to him a need for immediate surgery. He told the others it was necessary to now open up the patient's abdomen to identify and fix the issue.

As the team prepared for surgery, I noticed a second-year general surgery resident standing on the other side of the patient, next to the head surgeon. He had a very strange look on his face. He didn't look like he was going to pass out—although you'd see this happen from time to time. No, he looked more like he was in shock, or like he was holding in a big secret. I seemed to be the only one who noticed this. My attention went back to the patient, whose belly had by now been swabbed with iodine. Just as the head surgeon prepared to make the first cut, the resident across from me stopped him. The surgeon looked at him in surprise and obvious annoyance, waiting to hear what he had to say.

"I'm sorry sir, but it wasn't the patient," he began.

"What are you talking about?" the surgeon demanded.

"What I mean is you didn't smell the patient," the resident continued. He had turned an interesting shade of red. "It was me...um...I uh, well I passed gas," he finished. If the floor could have opened up, I think the poor resident would have jumped in.

The surgeon was furious. He had been seconds away from cutting down onto the patient. It was a very good thing the resident confessed, as embarrassing as it was for him. In the end, the patient did not end up having any sort of internal injury, which was lucky for him. He was sent for a CT scan, and the results confirmed this.

I'm not sure exactly what I took away from this besides a mildly inappropriate story that still gives me a chuckle whenever I think of it. Some stories you just can't make up.

CHAPTER 13

The Hit and Run

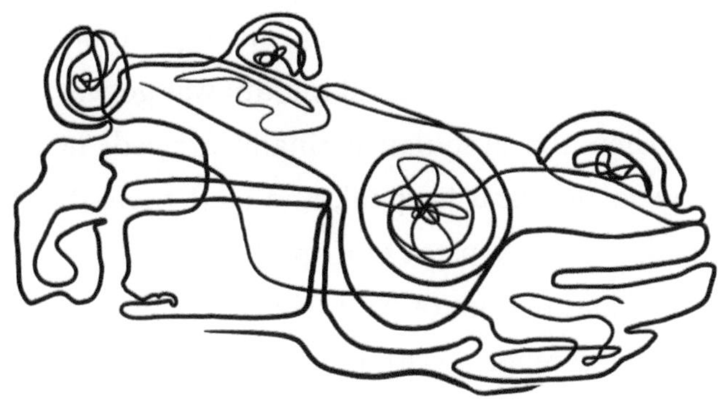

My next patient, Eduardo, came to me after a very bizarre series of events. While there are always two sides to any story, Eduardo seemed like a very authentic, open man. My accounting of what happened to him is based on what he told me.

Eduardo was a US citizen but had a business and home in Mexico. He would drive back and forth between his home in Southern California and Mexico regularly. One day while he was driving in Mexico,

Eduardo was in a major car accident. Someone had been driving on the wrong side of the road and ran into him, totalling his car. The impact of the collision knocked Eduardo out, and because he was not wearing his seatbelt, he went through the windshield. When he regained consciousness, he found himself on the pavement, surrounded by glass, and bleeding from several lacerations. Thankfully, some passersby saw him lying on the ground and called an ambulance. The driver and car that had hit him was gone.

When the ambulance finally arrived, he was taken to the local hospital, and staff there did the bare minimum to patch him up. He was still dirty and bloody, and in a lot of pain. He filled out a hospital admittance report, writing that he'd been the victim of a hit and run car accident. He remained in hospital for one or two days, and during that time, no MRIs, x-rays or CT scans were taken. When Eduardo told me this, I was shocked. If a patient was brought to me with the symptoms he described, I would have ordered several tests to determine whether he had sustained serious injuries. As I mentioned before, some Mexican citizens will forego treatment at a Mexican hospital and take their chances with the US immigration system because they believe they can receive better treatment and care here.

Eduardo was lucky to be alive, but he was in terrible shape and desperately needed treatment. He was still in a great deal of pain, and probably suffering from a concussion. He didn't really understand what had happened to him, or why nobody at the hospital had called his family to let them know what had happened. Then, on his second day in the hospital, the police showed up, put him in handcuffs, and took him to jail. Overwhelmed and in shock, he told me later that it felt like a bad dream, or a scene out of a movie.

He was informed by police that he had caused the accident, and that he had hurt other people and personal property. They told him he would not be permitted to receive proper medical care or to leave the prison until he had paid all the expenses. Eduardo had no idea what he was supposed to do. His first concern was about the excruciating pain he felt in his neck. He was worried that it might be broken. He knew he needed to get medical attention soon. He tried to explain that he had been hit by someone else, and not the other way around. He told the police that some people had found him lying on the ground, and the other car had taken off, but for some reason they refused to believe him. They kept insisting he pay them money for the damage he'd caused.

"I didn't cause the accident." He told them over and over again in both English and Spanish.

"That's what they all say," The policemen replied, then went about their business.

He asked to speak to a lawyer, and to be able to call his family, but his request was repeatedly denied. He was stuck there and completely at a loss for what to do next.

They probably figured he would eventually grow so desperate to leave that he would just pay the money. The trouble was, Eduardo really wasn't feeling well, and eventually he slipped to the floor and closed his eyes.

Somebody must have noticed him lying there and either found their conscience or got worried he might die and cause them unnecessary paperwork. Either way, they insisted that he needed immediate medical attention. He was brought back to the hospital, where staff finally performed some basic tests.

"Oh. It seems your neck is broken," The doctor told him, his voice tinged with surprise.

By this point, Eduardo didn't trust anything he was being told. His neck still hurt terribly but now he wondered whether the doctor was trying to shake him down for money the way the police had? Had the hospital and police worked together to try and extort him? He didn't care to know the answer, he just wanted to go home.

He didn't need to worry any longer that the hospital would try to hold him. Now that they knew he had a broken neck, they were suddenly very helpful in arranging for him to leave. Eduardo told me the doctors were so concerned about his neck fracture they didn't want to touch him and were worried about potential liability. His broken neck had turned out to be a blessing in disguise.

"Just get rid of the guy. Let him leave," he overheard one doctor say to another in the hall outside his room.

He was finally allowed to contact someone in the US for help, and they quickly made arrangements to pick him up and get him across the border.

It turned out that I had treated a friend of Eduardo's in the past, and they had referred him to me. By the time I saw him, about a week had passed since the time of his accident. When he came to my clinic, I ordered some x-rays and then a CT scan. The tests revealed he had a very serious fractured neck and it was unstable. And although he hasn't suffered a spinal cord injury yet, the neck fracture put him at very high risk for it happening. It was so bad that I told him he needed to be admitted to the hospital immediately. I was pretty sure he was going to need to have emergency surgery and I wanted him to get an MRI and some other tests right away. We also did an assessment to make sure there were no other injuries.

The results from the tests confirmed what I suspected; he would need emergency surgery. I explained to Eduardo that his neck was seriously broken and that he was at high risk for a spinal cord injury. He was very, very lucky he hadn't been paralyzed either at the time of the accident or afterwards, in the hospital or prison. The location of his injury put him at risk of permanently losing complete body function. I told him we needed to fix his neck, and he agreed. It required an operation from the front and back of his neck and involved the insertion of screws and rods to stabilize the area.

The surgery was a complete success and Eduardo did great. Within forty-eight hours he was able to leave the hospital and finally begin to put the ordeal behind him. I continued to follow up with him for another year to make sure he was healing properly and was getting physical therapy. After the year had passed, he had made a complete recovery and suffered no long-term damage.

During our last appointment just before he left my office, Eduardo said to me, "I appreciate everything you have done for me. If you and your wife are ever interested, you are welcome to stay my place in Mexico anytime." He went on to describe how beautiful the house was, and how picturesque the scenery.

I told him thank you for the kind offer, and said I'd let him know if we decided to take a vacation to Mexico.

He stood at the door to my office as we said goodbye. "It's funny," he said, looking thoughtful. "The house I own in Mexico is less than five minutes from where my accident happened."

"Funny," I echoed, wondering if he would ever feel safe driving that road again. I wasn't sure I'd ever take him up on his offer, but I knew the odds of us going would decrease exponentially if I shared Eduardo's story with my wife. I decided she didn't need to hear about *every* case I saw...

CHAPTER 14

Unique Farming Methods

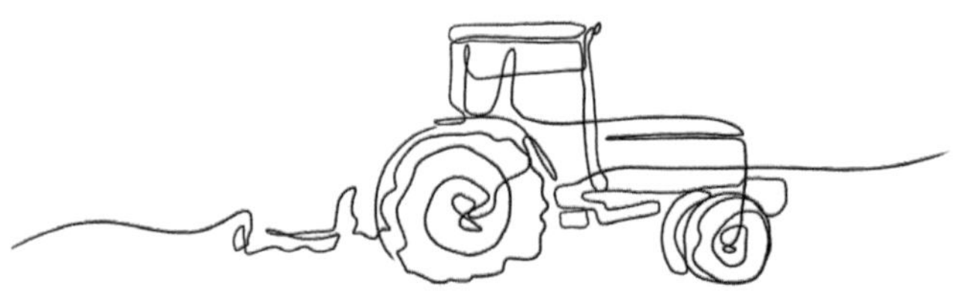

This next story is about a patient I helped while working in a hospital in San Diego. A badly injured patient had just been brought in from Mexico, and we were having a difficult time understanding what had happened despite the ambulance attendants' best efforts to explain. What they described sounded like something out of a movie rather than real life. It was only when I saw the patient that things finally started to make sense.

The patient was a Mexican farmer who had been injured while working his field. If you don't have a background in agriculture (or a patient who does), something you may not know is that at the end of a season, farmers will sometimes burn their fields. From what I understand, burning helps get rid of shrubs, roots, and crop residue—for example the fallen bits of hay and rice that are left in a field after harvesting. In these scenarios, farmers burn the field because they want to plant a new type of crop right away and don't want it contaminated by the old crop. Farmers also use burning as a method to control weeds and prevent disease and pests. But even a controlled burn must be closely supervised because there is always risk involved.

It was the end of the season and my patient had been tending to his family farm. He had recently finished harvesting his latest crop and had planned to till the soil then burn it so he could start a new crop. On the night of his accident, he had decided he was going to be a very efficient farmer and multitask. Alcohol, we would learn, had provided the inspiration for this particular genius idea. It was very dark out as the farmer drove the big cultivator machine across his field, with only a half empty bottle of liquor for company. A cultivator is a large piece of farming equipment with long teeth that turn in a rotary motion. It's used to break up the soil before planting. My patient's cultivator was self-propelling and was attached at the front of his tractor.

As he flicked the ashes of his cigarette onto the ground, he decided to light up the field behind him, reasoning that the tractor moved much faster than fire. Things seemed to be going according to plan until a rock got stuck in the rotor and the tractor stopped. Leaving the tractor running, the farmer stumbled over to try and get it unblocked before the fire caught up to him. You can imagine the panic he must have been feeling as he looked up to see flames racing towards him and his very expensive machine. Even sober, a person might have felt a little weak at the knees to see the fire approaching—and he was nowhere close to sober.

He picked up a stick and began poking at the rock, leaning in to better see what he was doing. He was so engrossed in his attempts to dislodge the rock that he lost his balance and fell headfirst into the rotor. The blades chopped up his scalp and skull and threw churned up soil and manure into the open wounds.

Luckily, it was a calm night and his screams carried across the field and were heard by a neighbor, who then saw the flames and came running over to help. Unfortunately, by the time the neighbor arrived, the fire had caught up to the farmer and he had suffered severe burns. The neighbor and the farmer's family were able to douse the fire and then brought him to the local hospital. When he arrived at the Mexican hospital, they realized his injuries were way beyond their ability to help, and they sent him over to us in San Diego, California.

When I saw him, he was in horrible shape; it was quite shocking actually. We immediately brought him to the emergency operating room, but I remember thinking there was no way this man was going to survive his injuries. We began irrigating his head wounds, literally trying to get the dirt out of his brain. After washing it, we were able to reconstruct his skull and tend to his burn wounds. It was a miracle, and a complete surprise for me, but the farmer managed to survive. The cultivator's blades missed his eyes, and although he did have quite a bit of scarring, and probably had some long-term brain damage, he would eventually be able to walk out of the hospital and return to his farm…truly a miracle.

CHAPTER 15

Freak Accident

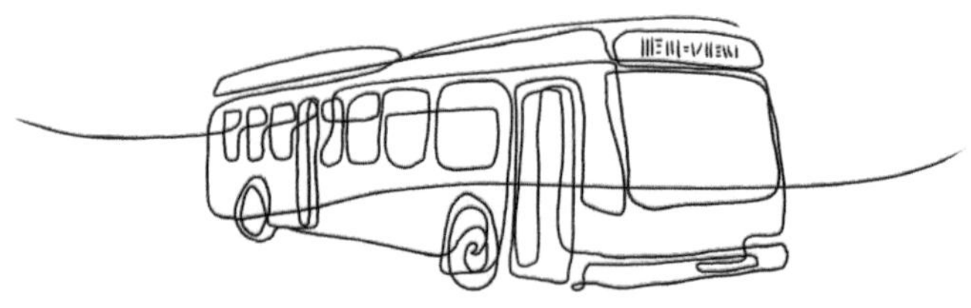

For those of you who have ever sat waiting for a bus, my next story might be quite frightening. A woman in her early forties was brought to us early one day. That morning I'd left home in a rush, grabbing only a quick cup of coffee on my way out the door. I was still in my residency. It had been a busy morning in the ER, and the smells of breakfast being served to patients throughout the hospital had awakened my appetite, making my stomach growl. I had planned to grab some fruit and maybe a bagel from the cafeteria to make up for my missed breakfast, but things had not slowed down enough for me to leave. This turned out to be a blessing in disguise.

Even before the stretcher bearing the patient's body burst through the doors of the ER, we could smell her burned flesh. I think the stomachs of everyone present—both patients and staff—gave a collective lurch as the dreadful smell of cooked flesh filled the room. Many of those who'd recently eaten went running for the exits, hands covering their mouths. In my periphery, I saw a couple of junior staff dabbing Vick's Vapor Rub on the inside of their masks. I didn't blame them, I was feeling a little green around the gills myself. Rubbing something pleasant smelling on our masks, such as vapor rub, wintergreen oil, or benzoin tincture, was a trick we used to handle bad odors. Over the years, I had become desensitized to most smells—you are exposed to so many, and so often, that you either get used to them or develop the ability to ignore them. I have to admit, however, that the permeating scent of this patient's charred, still-smoking flesh tested even my limits. My hunger pangs immediately disappeared and I had to force my stomach to stop its unsettled flip flopping.

The woman had been waiting for the bus she took every day to go to work. She had arrived early at her stop, as she often did, and had sat on the bench in the bus shelter to read her book while she waited. The bus shelter bench was covered by an awning that served to protect people from the elements during inclement weather. The bench and surrounding structure were metal, and the awning was attached to the structure with some metal poles. The bus shelter was also wired so that it would light up at night, presumably to make things safer for riders, and to make the stops more visible for bus drivers after dark.

In a bizarre turn of fate, the electricity in the shelter's awning short circuited while she sat there. Somehow the wires from the awning touched the metal of the supporting structure, shooting an electrical current down the poles and through the bench, causing the woman to be electrocuted. When the electrical current is strong enough, it can travel through a person's whole body exiting through the feet and going into the earth.

I'll never forget the sight and the smell of the woman. Her clothing in the area that had been in contact with the bench had been burned off her body. Much worse than her damaged clothes, the parts of her backside that had been touching the bench were completely cooked, right down to the bone. There was no muscle or fat remaining; it had completely melted off. The woman's heart had stopped from the electrocution, so our immediate priority was to try and get it restarted. Sadly, in spite of our best efforts, we were unable to get her heart pumping again. It was a traumatic experience for everyone involved. It wasn't just the smell; it was emotionally very difficult to see what had happened to her. Medical professionals often see things in their line of work that they wish they could unsee.

Following her death, the city did an investigation, and determined that it was in fact an accident. I was thankful when I heard she had been the only one at the bus stop, and no one else had been injured. The city's investigation found that it was not the first time this had happened in the US. Other people around the country had been electrocuted in similar accidents involving the same type of bus shelter awning, made by the same company. I could not understand how that company was still in business, or why they'd been allowed to continue making that type of shelter after the first time someone was electrocuted.

I have previously shared this story with my own family and friends. It may have been a freak accident, but it had happened more than once. My intention for sharing this very sad story is to let others know this sort of thing can happen. I haven't taken a bus in years, but if I ever do so again, I know without question that I would take my chances standing in the rain! Thankfully, this incident instigated serious investigations by the city and state authorities and led to an immediate reconstruction of these types of benches so hopefully it will never happen again.

CHAPTER 16

The Subtle Gunshot To The Brain

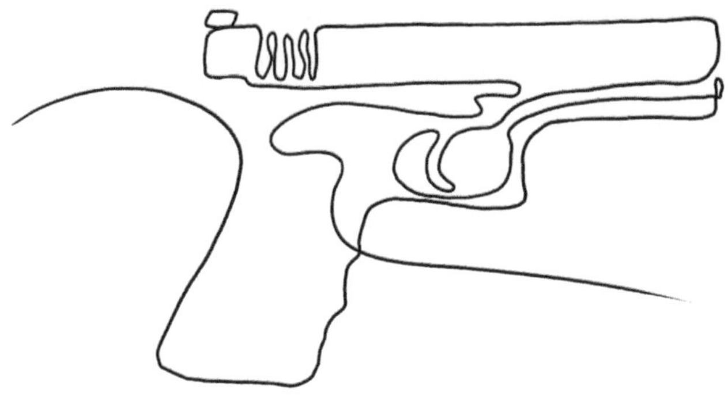

Gang violence is a sad reality in the US. Hospitals see a lot of people, both gang members and innocent bystanders, who are injured by this sort of violence. It's such a common occurrence that ER personnel receive gang identification training so they know what gang rivalries exist in their area and can recognize common gang identifiers, such as clothing and tattoos. Hospital staff have a series of safety and prevention protocols they must follow when gang members arrive at the hospital—whether they come in on a stretcher or sit in the waiting room. Situations can quickly become violent, and the goal of every hospital and medical professional is the safety and protection of human life.

On this particular day, a patient who was a gang member arrived in the emergency room. He was unwilling to provide a lot of details about what had happened, but we found out he had been involved in some sort of altercation with a rival gang. When he was brought in, hospital staff evaluated for his injuries and had found some cuts, abrasions and bruising but nothing dramatic. According to his evaluation report, he seemed to be generally doing okay. He was lying down on a hospital bed when I first came to see him. I remember walking over to him on his right side then introducing myself. He seemed surprised when I started speaking to him, and this was really strange. He was awake and alert, but it's like he hadn't seen me approach.

I was standing right next to him on the right beside his bed, and he had to turn dramatically to the right to be able to see me.

"I didn't see you there," he told me, looking startled. I was puzzled by this, but I continued talking to him and began to examine him. He told me that one of his abrasions, on the left side of his head really hurt. I was performing a more thorough neurological examination than the exam he'd first received. From my examination, I realized that he had a visual field cut, which means that he could not see out of a portion of his field of vision. He hadn't realized this, and the initial assessments had not picked up on it ether. It was very unusual because it should have been quite obvious to the patient that he was partially blind.

I asked him, "Have you had any problems with your vision lately?"

"No," he responded. As we talked, he had begun to realize something serious was wrong, and he started to feel scared. He told me he had never experienced anything like this before.

I continued my examination, checking his ability to smell and hear, as well as a number of other neurological tests. I could not find any clues that might help me figure out why he had this visual field cut. I began examining his head, and noticed he had a very small cut on the back left side. The area where the cut was located is called the occipital region.

"How did you get this little cut?" I asked him.

"I don't know but my head really hurts in that spot," he answered.

I said to my team "Let's get a CT scan of his head to see what's going on."

They asked me why he needed a CT scan, when the report as well indicated he was not suffering from any serious injuries.

I explained about the visual field cut and the painful abrasion I'd found on the back of his head. I told them I was concerned he might have a deeper injury. When the results of the CT scan came back, it showed he had a bullet lodged in his brain.

The unique thing about the occipital lobe on the left side of the brain is that if you injure that area, it affects the right side of both of your eyes. So the right half of your left eye, and the right half of your right eye will be impaired. This explained why the patient could not see me when I approached him on his right side.

It was odd to me that the patient had not even realize he'd been shot in his head. At the very least he should have noticed the loud pop sound that came from the gun when it was fired. We would later learn that the bullet was a small caliber, but even so, I would have expected to see more bleeding in that area. He was lucky because aside from the visual impairment, he did not suffer any other brain injury. While upset that he had permanently lost a portion of his vision, he did seem grateful to be alive.

We did surgery to remove the bullet, and the operation was a complete success. A short time later he was discharged from the hospital. I'd like to think his near-death experience might have caused him to re-evaluate some of his life choices.

CHAPTER 17

The Pot Lid

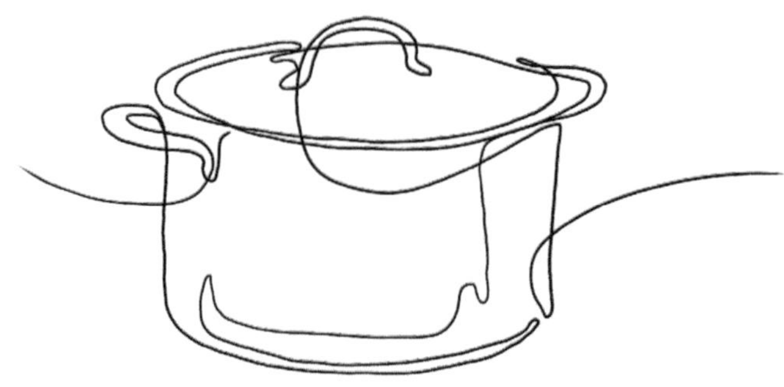

As a doctor, I meet people from all walks of life. In my many years of practice, I've treated my share of interesting patients. Some patients are fascinating because of their conditions, and sometimes it is their disposition or other personal attributes that make them stand out. I strive to always keep an open mind and be respectful of my patients' personal experiences and perspectives. At the heart of what I do lies a deep-seated desire to help people.

Patients will sometimes bring things with them to their appointments. These "things" tend to fall into three categories. A patient might bring a physical therapy appliance, such as a brace or orthotic device, or maybe a cushion to sit on. If I'm doing a consult for a child, they might be carrying a security blanket or stuffed animal when their parents bring them in. This is not unusual. Some patients bring gifts, such as cookies or flowers, as a kind of post-operative thank you. While unnecessary, it's a thoughtful gesture and I'm always touched when a patient does this. Upon occasion I've had people bring a personal support animal to their appointments. Although a rare occurrence, I've never had a problem with this. But by far the most...uncommon...item a patient has ever brought to an appointment is a pot lid.

A man came to see me a few years back for a first-time consult. His name was Boris, and he was in his mid-sixties. He had been suffering from a sore back and wanted to know if there was anything I could do for him. When Boris walked into my office, I could tell something was wrong immediately. He walked with care, and as he sat down he did so in the way people often do when they are in pain. He gripped the arm rest of his chair with one hand and let himself slowly ease into it. He had a bit of difficulty, because his other hand was gripping a large, mangled pot lid. I was intrigued and waited for him to explain why he'd brought the lid with him. I imagined it would be a good story.

Rather than explaining it however, Boris carefully set the lid down on the chair next to him and gave it a pat. I began the appointment with the usual pleasantries and asked him to tell me what had brought him in. While we were chatting, I found myself a bit distracted by the pot lid. It was difficult not look at it, and I had to consciously remind myself to maintain eye contact as Boris went through his health history. It was the kind of lid you would use to cover a large spaghetti pot. Bent and dented, it had clearly seen better days. Boris was oblivious to my inquisitive gaze, and in no hurry to explain the pot lid's significance.

"My back hurts all the time," he told me. "I've tried different medicines, but they don't take away the pain. I've tried different kinds of physical therapy and so far nothing has worked." He'd put a hand on the lid while he was talking and kept it there.

I started to wonder if the lid was some sort of comfort object for Boris. Maybe it was something he carried around with him all the time. I'd seen people bring in a favorite old quilt, or weighted blanket to their appointments. Sometimes they brought photos, worry beads or their rosary. Parents sometimes brought pacifiers, toys or fidget spinners for their children to keep them occupied during the talking part of our appointments. I'd seen people holding good luck charms, crystals and rocks from time to time. None of these things had distracted me the way the large pot lid on the seat across from me did now.

"—I'd started to think nothing was going to help me Dr. Ozgur..." Boris said.

Please don't let him tell me he thinks the pot lid is helping him, I thought, catching myself looking at the lid and correcting the direction of my gaze once again.

"Lucille said you were the best, and that's why I'm here." Boris was looking at the chair and its occupant beside him as he said this.

Dear God, he thinks the lid can talk, I thought, realizing Boris could be suffering from some sort of psychological disorder.

"That was very kind of Lucille," I replied politely, looking briefly at the chair beside him, then back at him again.

"She told me you treated her last year for back troubles," he continued.

"Erm...*Lucille* told you this?" I asked, feeling a bit puzzled.

"Yes, she saw you last year." He clarified.

Upon further questioning, I realized with relief Lucille had indeed been a patient of mine last year.

When did your back issues begin?" I asked him.

Boris told me the pain had begun about eighteen months ago.

We were about fifteen minutes into the appointment by now, and Boris was oblivious to my now-burning curiosity about the pot lid.

"Tell me what happened," stealing another quick glance. I could not seem to stop myself.

"Well, you know, politics in this country have been just crazy the last few years," Boris began.

"Yes," I said, nodding. *Come on Boris, what's the deal with the pot lid?* My mind urged.

"Well, there's been lots of arguing back and forth about politics and so forth," Boris said with a frown. He patted the lid absently as he spoke.

The political climate in the US had been quite tense over the past few years, and many people had rather polarized views on the topic. I had heard of divided households, where entire families were torn apart because of politics. It was very sad.

"Yes," I repeated, leaning forward now to signal my interest and encouragement. I wondered if Boris had driven to this appointment with the pot lid on the passenger seat beside him, and whether he'd strapped it in with the seat belt. I covered my mouth with my hand and cleared my throat to cover my smile.

Thankfully, Boris didn't notice. "It was about a year and a half ago, and I had invited some friends over for dinner," he began. We were all standing around the kitchen and I was finishing up the sauce for the spaghetti," he said.

My ears perked up when he mentioned the spaghetti. This *had* to be the link to the pot lid.

"We got into a big argument about politics, and it got pretty heated." He added.

Did he hit someone with the lid? I wondered, fighting the urge to look at the lid again.

"I guess I got so frustrated, I just couldn't help it." He continued.

He hit someone, I thought. I hoped the person wasn't hurt. The lid was seriously banged up.

"Well, I lost my temper and just got real upset." Boris said.

Hmmm... maybe the lid is a weapon. The thought was a little unnerving. I tried not to think about the possibility of my own head adding another dent to the lid if he didn't like what I said.

"I don't even remember what our fight was about." He said, looking thoughtful.

"Okay," I said, feeling my right eyelid beginning to twitch.

"Well I guess I grabbed the pot lid and I just slammed it onto the kitchen counter as hard as I could." He finished. Then he picked up the pot lid and held it out for me to examine more closely.

I felt something relax inside me, the eye twitch ceasing immediately.

Boris must have used quite a bit of force when he slammed the pot lid down on the counter. He was suffering from a significant spinal fracture in his back, and this explained the pain he was experiencing. Luckily, he did not require surgery, and I was able to treat him conservatively. I recommended physical therapy, a back brace, and a couple other treatment options, and in a relatively short period of time, his pain completely went away.

This patient experience is one that still makes me laugh. One of the things I love most about my job, besides being able to help people, is the interaction with my patients. Every one of them has a compelling story that deserves to be heard. Some, like Boris, just take a little longer to get to the punch line.

CHAPTER 18

Spine Envy

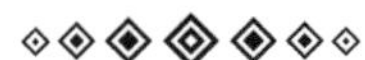

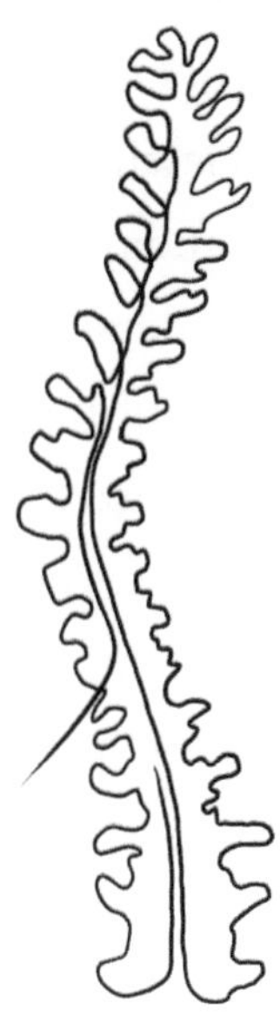

This story is about a woman in her late fifties who came to see me about the possibility of having spine surgery. The woman had been to see several different physicians who all told her she had a typical chronic spine degeneration as well as a type of scoliosis that was probably genetic. She had been treated conservatively, meaning she had not had surgery for her condition. Instead, she'd done physical therapy and had received treatment by pain specialists, but she felt unsatisfied with the results. She told me she was interested in exploring possible surgical options to fix her spine issues.

During our appointment, she admitted she was at her wits end and could not handle the pain any longer. I'd spent some time reviewing her patient file and had also asked her some standard questions to give me a more comprehensive understanding of her case. She started asking questions of her own on the topic of genetics, which I found puzzling at first. She didn't seem to accept what I was saying when I told her that surgery was unfortunately not an option for her.

"Your best option is to continue with the treatment options your previous physician suggested." I told her. She looked at the floor and shook her head.

Rather than responding to what I had said, she asked me more questions relating to genetics. I responded with much the same messaging that I'd used before, hoping it would sink in. When she finally realized she wasn't going to get what she wanted from me, she asked about the possibility of having a spine transplant.

"We can transplant hearts, livers, and other body parts, so can't you exchange my spine with a healthier one?" She demanded.

"That's an interesting question," I said. It was not the first time someone had asked me this, and I could understand why the question came up. "Unfortunately spinal transplants are not possible yet," I explained. "In spite of the incredible advances in modern medicine, we're just not there." I spoke for a few minutes about the factors that made it impossible.

"But can you transplant my spine?" she asked, looking at me like I'd been speaking Greek for the last ten minutes.

"No," I said.

"Why not?" she demanded, an edge of frustration in her voice.

"The spine is too integrated into our body," I told her calmly. "The spinal cord goes through the frame of our skeleton, so we cannot cut it and reattach it." I felt compassion for her and understood some of her frustration. It was difficult to learn there was no perfect solution to her spine problem. I wanted to be respectful of her questions and let her know I took them seriously. She continued to press me on the matter, but my answers remained the same. I had the growing sense this woman was not used to taking no for an answer.

Finally, she asked, "Well, why can't you? I already have somebody in mind who could give me their spine."

This caught me off guard. "Excuse me?" I asked, in spite of myself. I couldn't help wondering what she was talking about.

"Well, my mother is really old," she began, looking intently at me now. "She's probably going to die soon anyway, and she won't need her spine," she said matter-of-factly.

Mistaking my silence for interest rather than shock, she continued. "Since she's not going to need her spine for long anyway, I can probably convince her to give it to me. Then you can transplant it into me."

I wondered if one of my colleagues had set this up as an elaborate hoax. I felt unease and confusion bubbling up inside of me and as I looked at her, I realized she was completely serious. I immediately schooled my face and let her finish talking.

The woman told me her mother was in her eighties, and because they shared a partial genetic structure, she figured her body wouldn't reject her mother's spine. "We share the same blood and are from the same family," she reasoned. "Plus she does yoga three times a week. She has beautiful posture and a lovely, straight spine."

"Are you serious?" I asked, incredulous.

Mistaking my horror for interest, she continued to share her perspective on the matter.

"You're saying that if spinal transplant surgery were possible—which it isn't—you'd volunteer your mother to give us her spine and put it in you?" I asked.

"Yes," she answered.

"After she died you mean?" I asked.

"Well she'd be dead eventually I suppose." the woman responded cryptically.

I struggled to hold back my shock. I explained that what she'd suggested was simply not currently possible. As delicately as I could, I told her that not only would it not be safe, but that it was not ethical either. I recommended that we deal with the spine that she had and told her my team and I would do the very best that we could for her.

She eventually accepted what I was saying and agreed to my proposed treatment plan as well. I was pleased that I'd be able to help her, and I hoped this put an end to her dreams of one day harvesting her mother's spine.

CHAPTER 19

Carpenter's Headache

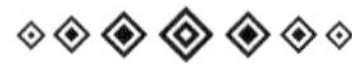

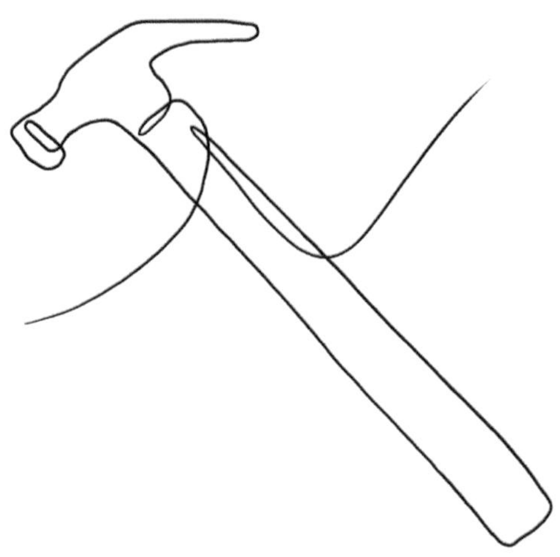

A carpenter by the name of Joe came to see me about a persistent headache he'd had for about two weeks. Joe was a skilled craftsman who worked in the construction industry, building houses, doing things like installing floor beams, walls and roofing systems. It was a very physical job, and he did a lot of wood cutting, measuring and joining of wood products. When his headaches began to interfere with his ability to work, he went to see his primary care doctor. The doctor conducted a standard series of tests but had been unable to figure out what was causing the headaches, so he had recommended Joe come see me.

When I first met Joe, I immediately noticed a small scar between his upper lip and his nose. I asked him about it, and he told me he cut it when he'd slipped and hit his face at work a couple weeks ago. I made a mental note but didn't think much about it. I did a physical examination, checking Joe's vision, hearing, the movement of his face, and various other things during the appointment, and everything appeared normal. I could not find any physical reason to explain his headaches, so I sent him for a CT scan. I was shocked when I saw the results.

Joe had a nail in his head. When I talked to him about it, he was surprised. He'd had no idea it was there. It turned out, on the day he'd hit his face at work, he'd been using a pneumatic nail gun. He had been running it along a piece of wood when it had recoiled. This type of tool has the same sort of recoil as a regular gun, and at some point, he had gotten too close. The nail gun must have turned somehow and hit him in the face, and when it hit him, he must have pulled the trigger. Due to the speed at which this tool fires, Joe did not realize what had happened. He probably thought his injury and the pain where the nail had entered had been caused by the impact off the kickback. He was incredibly lucky that it had not caused more severe or long-term damage.

In addition to the CT scan, I ordered an MRI to pinpoint the trajectory of the nail and surrounding structures. The nail had shot up through his sinuses into his brain. We scheduled surgery and were able to safely remove the nail. The procedure was a success. Joe made a complete recovery, and the headaches went away.

When I tell this story, people are often amazed that he did not realize he'd shot himself. Similar to the story titled "Gang Violence," where a gang member is shot in the back of the head but does not realize it, when a projectile object is very small, it can sometimes be missed. In cases like this, patients will come in seeking relief for a particular symptom, and I will often discover the root cause is something completely different or unexpected. In my practice, I have learned to pay attention to even the smallest details, because many times it's those seemingly minor things that wind up being the key to solving a patient's case. When I meet with patients, I typically ask them to retell their medical history, and urge them to be as detailed as possible. As they say, "the devil is in the details." Sometimes the solution to a problem exists there as well.

CHAPTER 20

Tragic Consequences

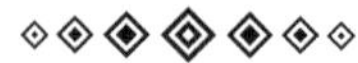

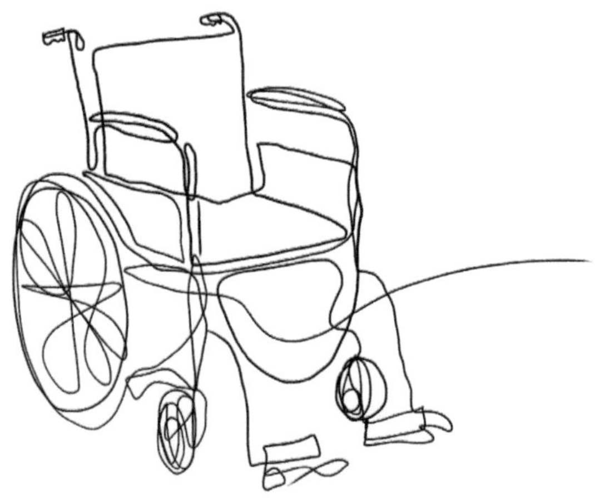

An off-duty police officer was driving home after work one evening, when the events of this next story unfolded. The man had stopped to pick up his six-year-old-son on his way home. The child was in the back seat, and for some reason he did not have his seatbelt on; it's possible the child managed to unbuckle himself. His son slid down onto the floor and found the man's duty gun, which the man had left there after he finished work. To make matters worse, the man had not unloaded the gun or even bothered to put the safety on. I'm sure you can see where this is going.

While the child was on the floor of the car playing with the gun, it went off. Thankfully the man's son had not been pointing the gun at himself, and he was unharmed. Unfortunately, the gun had been pointed at the back of the man's seat when it discharged, and the bullet ripped through the seat and lodged in his dad's spine. The man had somehow managed to stop the car safely and get help.

When the man was brought into the hospital he was paralyzed. We quickly examined him and did a CT scan, then rushed him into surgery. Truth be told, the man was lucky to be alive. Unfortunately, although we were able to remove the bullet, clean up the area and close up the wound, the bullet had damaged his spinal cord in a way that could not be repaired. There was nothing more we could do. The man was permanently paralyzed from the waist down.

The boy had been brought in with his father, and his wails filled the ER. He was terrified, not grasping what had happened, fearing he had "hurt his daddy." I worked with a grim heaviness in my heart, as did the rest of the medical team. It was a relief when his mother arrived to get him, but the echo of his sobs stayed with me long after he was taken home.

It was a tragedy on two fronts. On the one hand, it was terrible what had happened to the man. His career as a police officer was over and he would never walk again. But it was also terrible to think about the long-term psychological impact this accident would have on his son. The boy would grow up knowing that this accident was responsible for putting his father in a wheelchair.

It's easy to become desensitized to things we see in our everyday environment. Consider my job as an example. Some people get squeamish at the sight of blood, and yet it doesn't bother me at all. I see it every day, and for me it is simply a substance that flows through the body carrying oxygen and nutrients. For that police officer, guns were something he saw and handled every day. It was simply a tool of his job, and because he was comfortable around them, he may have dropped his guard a little bit.

CHAPTER 21

Assaulted with a Frozen Tuna

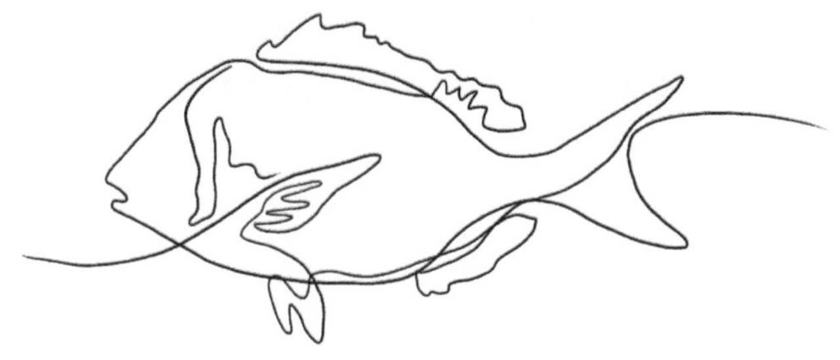

Things can happen very quickly in the Emergency Room of a hospital, and the effective exchange of information between health service providers is critical. Sometimes before a doctor meets a patient, the attending nurse will give a quick one-liner to explain the most important thing the doctor should know about the patient. For example, they'll say, "This is a thirty-year-old man who was in a car accident."

In this story, as I was hurrying over to see a patient who had recently arrived in the ER, a nurse gave me a most unusual one-liner. "Thirty-eight-year-old man assaulted with a frozen tuna." She said it with a perfectly straight face. This sounded fishy to me.

When I met the patient he was disoriented but confirmed he had indeed been walloped in the head with a large, frozen tuna. A CT scan revealed he had a skull fracture as well as a hematoma on the side of his head. His condition was potentially life threatening, and it required immediate surgery. We had to go in and remove the blood clot and repair the skull fracture. It was only after the surgery that we learned the full story.

One of the things I love about living in Southern California is its large coast line. It is very picturesque. Tourism is a big industry here, and there are a lot of fishing boat operators who will take tourists out on multi-day trips. On these excursions, people have the opportunity to do deep sea fishing. Because they go quite far and are gone for so long, the boats are equipped with large refrigerators and chest freezers, which are used to store any fish that is caught to keep it from spoiling. At the end of the trip, the fish is taken out of the freezers and put on the deck so people can take pictures with their catch and then clean the fish before arriving at the dock.

In this particular case, my patient and his girlfriend had gone out on an excursion and had caught several tuna on their trip. It sounded like three days in close quarters had not brought out the best in this couple, and on the last day, as the crew took out the now-frozen tuna, the couple got into a heated argument over something or other. My patient estimated the tuna was almost three feet long, which is roughly the length of a baseball bat. Their argument had intensified, and in a moment of passion, his girlfriend picked up the tuna and swung it at him, managing to hit him squarely on the side of his head.

The surgery was a success, and my patient suffered no long-term damage. During his time in the hospital, the man's girlfriend was noticeably absent. Although curious, I was not about to fish for more details. It was none of my business.

CHAPTER 22

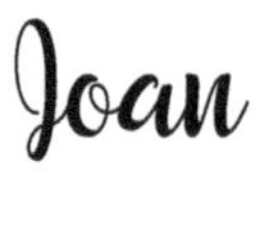

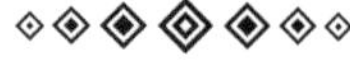

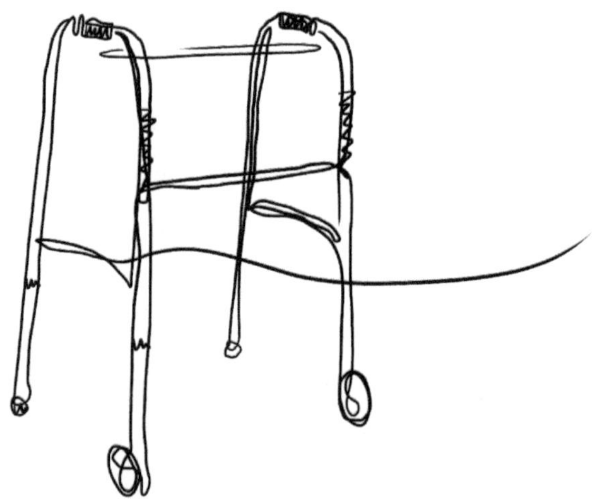

My next patient, Joan, was a sweet woman in her early eighties. Joan had a type of cyst in her back that was attached to a joint in her spine. The cyst was pressing on the nerves in her spine, causing severe pain to radiate from her back all the way down her legs. Her problem was easily fixable with a relatively minor spine surgery. When I offered her the surgery, she was ecstatic. Her life had been greatly impacted by the pain caused by the cyst, and she'd been unable to do many of the things she loved, such as swimming, playing the piano, and socializing with friends. The problem wasn't that her condition was inoperable; it was simply that before she met me, no surgeon had been willing to perform the operation because of her age.

In my practise I see a lot of older patients who have very common spine problems that can be fixed. The unfortunate reality for these older patients is that a lot of doctors out there just look at their age and say, "Oh you're too old to undergo spine surgery." Many doctors see a patient's advanced age as a liability, so instead of a simple surgery, they will often recommend a more conservative approach to treatment. For example, they will suggest physical therapy, medications, and/or narcotics to deal with the problem.

A lot of older patients come to see me to explore minimally invasive options, such as microscopic surgery, which is a smaller, safer, and easier route compared to more traditional spinal surgery. The risk of complications for this kind of surgery is minimal, as is the recovery time for most patients. Often the results of this kind of surgery are immediate and profoundly noticeable.

Joan's procedure involved removing the cyst and cleaning up the area around it. Her surgery went great, and she was up and walking easily within hours. Best of all, her symptoms were completely gone. She was very grateful to have her life back, and grateful to me for performing the surgery. It did my heart good to see her looking so happy.

Medical science has come a long way, and it is remarkable how much we can now do to help people. If a patient is otherwise healthy, the fact that they are older doesn't preclude them from surgery. Sometimes elderly people wind up being the healthier patients, for example when you compare them to a sixty-year-old obese patient with heart disease who smokes and drinks. I would choose to do surgery on the healthy eighty-year-old.

Helping people like Joan reminds me of why I love what I do. If you'd like to see a video of Joan's story, you can find it on YouTube at:
https://www.youtube.com/watch?v=dfQxBI6t0e0

CHAPTER 23

A Mother's Intuition

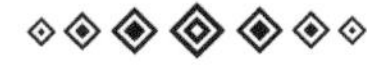

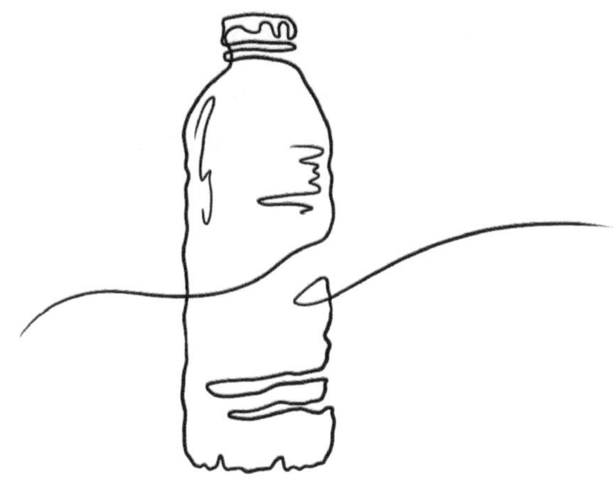

My next patient was a really sweet young lady named Lucy, whom, I discovered, was suffering from a complex spinal problem. Additionally, Lucy had Down syndrome, which is a genetic condition caused by abnormal cell division during the development of a fetus in the womb. It's also known as trisomy 21, and people who have this condition carry an extra chromosome. Physical and intellectual characteristics associated with Down syndrome include growth delays and mental disabilities.

Lucy's mother, Jennifer, told us that although Lucy was physically twenty-one, intellectually she was more like a ten-year-old. Lucy was in a wheelchair when I met her and was completely dependent on her mother to take care of her. Jennifer had dedicated her life to taking care of her daughter, and the bond between them was obvious to me. Although Lucy was nonverbal, she was able to interact with her mother in other ways. It was very interesting for me to watch Jennifer and Lucy communicate. Because she was nonverbal, it was not always clear to me what Lucy was communicating, but she and her mother had a very good connection.

Jennifer had brought her daughter in because she felt Lucy had a neck problem.

"How do you know she has a neck problem?" I asked. I could see that Lucy had a lot of dysfunctions already, so it wasn't clear to me what was new and what might have been a pre-existing condition.

"Well, movement wise, she's the same." Jennifer answered. "But I just know something is wrong. Call it a mother's intuition."

"Okay, so how do you know something is wrong?" I asked, looking for clues that could help me diagnose Lucy's problem.

"Well, for the past two months, whenever Lucy wants water, she wants it to be cold." Jennifer said.

"Is this unusual?" I probed.

"Yes, it is," Jennifer answered, looking at her daughter then at me. "She used to only want her water at room temperature." She said.

My mind was running through a compendium of conditions that might include temperature sensitivity as a symptom. I needed to know more. "What do you think the significance is of the cold water?" I asked.

"Well, she takes the cold water bottle I give her and she puts it on the back of her neck," she said.

This would make sense if Lucy had pain in her neck, I thought. "It sounds like she might be using the water bottle as a sort of makeshift icepack," I told Jennifer.

Jennifer agreed, looking relieved that I was taking her concern seriously.

I did a complete workup on Lucy, then sent her for a CT scan and some MRIs. I was hoping the tests would reveal the source of her problem. It must have been very stressful for Jennifer to sense that something might be wrong and know her daughter could not clearly communicate what it was. As a parent, I could empathize with her.

The tests revealed Lucy had a very complicated problem. It was no wonder she had neck pain. Her problem was actually quite serious, and Lucy was at risk of potentially becoming paralyzed if it was not fixed. The area between the top of her spine and the base of her skull, which is known as the occipital-cervical junction, had become unstable. This can happen with patients who have certain types of Down syndrome. It is a type of connective tissue problem where the spine and other parts of the body can become too lax, and it starts moving abnormally.

The area between Lucy's skull and cervical spine (neck) had become so unstable that it was essentially collapsing in on itself and pinching the spinal cord. This would undoubtedly result in severe neck pain at the very least. It was pretty amazing that Jennifer had picked up on the problem, and it spoke volumes about the loving attention she gave her daughter.

Now that we had identified the problem, we had to consider how we were going to resolve it. The surgical fix for this problem would be very complicated for anybody. But things were even more complex in Lucy's case. Not only would the surgery be difficult, but the recovery would also be challenging. I explained my proposed solution to Jennifer, and she was fully supportive of doing it if it meant preventing paralysis and alleviating her daughter's pain in the long term.

I recommended she communicate to Lucy what we were planning to do. I wanted Lucy to understand that her recovery was going to be arduous. Watching them interact, I could see some sort of understanding pass between them and felt that Lucy now had some comprehension of what would be involved.

The surgery itself was quite rare. It involved fusing Lucy's skull to her neck to stabilize it. I had to put plates and screws in to fuse things together. It was very difficult because a part of her neck bone was pushing from the front to the back part of her spinal cord in a hard-to-reach area. The challenge was that I couldn't reach it from the typical neck area because the location was so high. I had to go through the back of her mouth to the tip of her spine and remove a part of the bone. I then had to close things up and fuse the back of her skull to her neck. The surgery took eight hours to complete.

Lucy was amazing throughout her recovery. Anyone else going through such a complicated surgery and recovery would have complained because of the pain and physical limitations. Knowing her mental age, it would have been perfectly understandable if

Lucy had become upset, withdrawn or frightened. Oftentimes, children who go through surgery can become frightened of their doctors, associating them with the negative aspects of their hospital experience. Lucy had a naturally happy disposition, and she seemed to love everyone. It was a long road to recovery, requiring months in the acute rehab unit (ARU) after she was discharged from the hospital, but Lucy never once complained. She and her mother made a great team, and they both seemed to just take things one day at a time. We treated Lucy with medications and physical therapy as much as we could, and she slowly but surely got better.

She quickly became a favorite among hospital and ARU staff. People were wonderful with her, and through it all she was very cooperative, collaborative and sweet tempered. I am very happy to report that she made an amazing recovery and healed perfectly. She no longer wanted to hold cold water bottles against her neck, which told us her pain was gone. As a surgeon I'm supposed to remain impartial, but Lucy's resilience made a big impression on me, and it brought tears to my eyes when I finally saw her smile.

Jennifer told me Lucy's dream had always been to visit Disneyland. She loved Disney princesses and had always wanted to meet one in real life. Sometime after

Lucy had fully recovered and was able to return home, she and her mother were invited to go to Disneyland. There are several charitable organizations that work with people who have Down Syndrome, and one of them had arranged for Lucy and her mother to go to Disneyland. What made the trip extra special for Lucy was the fact they were able to arrange for Lucy to meet several of the Disney princesses and get a picture with them. Lucy and her mother came to see me after their trip, and they brought me a picture of Lucy with the princesses. Lucy's smile, as she stood in the middle of all the princesses, lit up her entire face. The picture was autographed, and on the back Lucy's mother had written a warm note of thanks to me for helping Lucy get better.

I blamed my watering eyes on allergies, but her words and their sweet gesture touched my heart deeply. I told Jennifer she and her daughter were an inspiration to me, and I meant it. I was glad to have been able to use my skills to help improve Lucy's quality of life.

CHAPTER 24

Hat's Off

◇◈◈◈◈◈◇

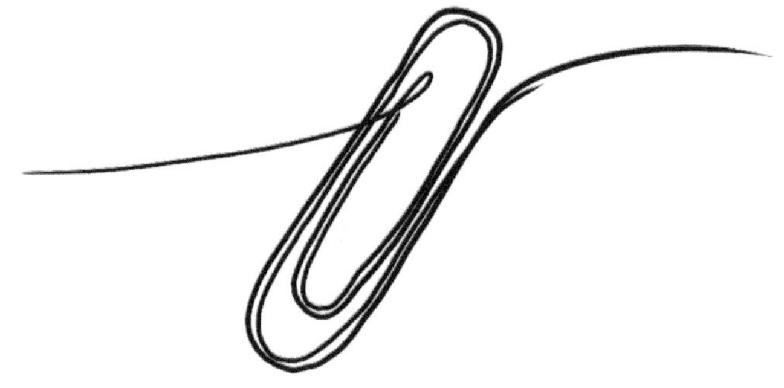

Similar to Lucy in the story "A Mother's Intuition," the patient in this next story had Down syndrome. In addition to Down syndrome however, Emanuel was severely autistic. These conditions, as well as some others, had created significant development delays in Emanuel. I first met him when he was thirteen years old, when his mother brought him in. Like Lucy in "A Mother's Intuition," he was nonverbal, but had a way of connecting with his mother.

Emanuel had frequent tics and repetitive mannerisms; he was always shaking or fidgeting or doing other things that involved movement of some kind. The reason his mother had wanted a neurosurgeon to see him was because he had injured his head. When I first saw Emanuel I could not see his injury because he had a hat on. His mother explained that he always wore it. Not wanting to upset Emanuel, I told her this was fine for now.

His mom explained that one of his mannerisms was to take a paperclip and repetitively scratch it against something. Typically it was a table or other piece of furniture, so this had not been of great concern for her. What she hadn't realized, because he always wore the hat, was that he'd begun to scratch his head with the paperclip. He had managed to cut through the skin on his head, using the paperclip to slowly scratch back and forth in the same spot, over and over again. Not only had he cut the skin, but over time he had actually worn down the bone and gotten through his skull. He had scratched it so deep in fact, that he had cut through the dura, which is the covering of the brain and gotten to the point where he had reached the surface of the brain.

I was amazed that his mother had not noticed the injury before now. It's possible his hair had covered it, or he had kept his hat on the whole time. She had only noticed the problem when his head began to leak clear fluid. The fluid that was leaking out was actually spinal fluid, which covers the brain and the spinal cord. When she realized what he'd done and contacted her son's primary care physician, he'd recommended they come through the ER and see me immediately.

Luckily the wound hadn't become infected yet, and it was a relatively straightforward surgery to close it up. We had to open Emanuel's scalp and then open a small portion of the skull so we could repair that damaged dura. After that it was a simple matter of closing everything up properly and sealing the hole that he had created by stitching up the skin. The surgery was a success, and Emanuel came through it without any complications.

What proved to be very difficult was keeping Emanuel from picking at his stitches. He began to play with them almost immediately after he woke up from surgery, and it was hard to deter him. We were concerned about him eventually cutting through or ripping out the stitches and the site becoming infected. We tried several things to distract him, but none of them worked. His mother was at her wits end.

We came up with an interesting trick that involved Steri-Strips and Dermabond, which ended up being the solution to this problem. Steri-Strips are little butterfly-shaped bandages that are sometimes used for closing a cut. They basically look like a sticker. If somebody has a cut somewhere, you put this bandage on at a ninety-degree angle and it just helps pull the skin together. Dermabond works like glue, and on some cuts it's used instead of stitches. We just glue across a cut or wound and seal it closed.

As the saying go, "necessity is the mother of all invention." Concerned that if he kept playing with his stitches his head might become infected, him mom and I came up with a plan to create "decoys" for him. We began putting the little Steri-Strips on his arms and legs. We also added little drips of the Dermabond glue to his skin as well. Because the glue sat superficially on his skin it was safe and would not hurt or harm him in any way. Thankfully, the strips and glue were enough to distract him. When it was time for him to leave the hospital, I gave a package of the strips and a tube of the glue to his mom. I told her to periodically put one or the other on one of his arms or legs so he would fixate on that instead of his head.

Our plan worked perfectly. Emanuel ended up recovering completely from his injury and surgery, much to his mother's and my relief. From then on, his mother was extra vigilant and made sure he never scratched his head, or anywhere else, with sharp objects again.

CHAPTER 25

If You Thought Your Day Was Crappy...

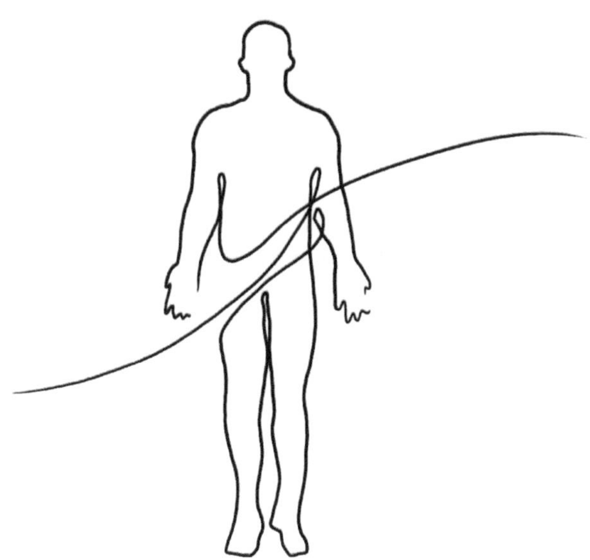

As we age, we go through changes in our bodies. For example, our tissues start to sag, and our ligaments get softer. This happens to varying degrees depending on the person. Another thing that can happen as we age is that our colon can get twisted on the inside. This can be dangerous, as the twisted area can turn the colon into a bit of a balloon, which can rupture. When the colon twists like this in one particular area it is called a sigmoid volvulus.

I was working as an intern on the general surgery service when I met this next patient, who was a woman in her eighties. The woman had an extra stretchy segment of colon, which caused the sigmoid part of her colon to twist sometimes. Every time it happened, she would get constipated and gassy, and because it prevented her from being able to pass any stool, she would experience severe abdominal pain.

Each time this would happen to her, she would come to the hospital to have it untwisted. It was a straightforward procedure, and she would go home immediately afterwards. The way we would treat cases like hers was to use what's called a rigid sigmoidoscope. It's a tube that's inserted into the colon via a person's bottom end. It has a camera so you can see what you are doing; it's similar to doing a colonoscopy, except that the tube is more rigid. The tube has to be inserted very carefully, but it's rigidness enables it to help untwist the colon. This is a little gross to describe, but when you untwist the colon, the contents of the bowels will immediately evacuate in a forceful way. Think of a shotgun going off and you'll get the picture. If you don't expect this, you will get covered with it.

In this particular case, I knew the woman's history from hearing the other residents talk about it. I knew that whoever was going to be doing the procedure would want to have a full gown, gloves and a face shield on. You'd want to be prepared and come completely protected. Now remember I was just an intern at the time doing a rotation in general surgery. The senior resident on this case was a more senior general surgery resident and he was years ahead of me in his training. He had not met the woman before and was not familiar with her case.

The woman was already prepped and ready to go when the senior resident entered the room where the procedure was to take place.

"There's something you should know about this patient—" I began.

"I know everything I need to know," the senior resident cut in.

"It's just that you might not be prepared—" I said.

"I think I know a little more than you do." He said curtly, cutting me off again.

I kept trying to explain to him that given this patient's situation, he might want to, well, um...prepare himself for what was to come, but he wouldn't let me finish. My concern was that he was only wearing his scrubs and a regular hospital mask. He continued to get increasingly annoyed. "Shut up! I know what I'm doing," he snapped.

"Okay, I was just trying to—" I began.

He held up a hand and stared at me hard. He seemed determined to handle this one on his own.

The senior resident positioned the woman on her side, similar to the way we would if we were doing a colonoscopy. I was at the front of her, near her head, and was responsible for holding her in the correct position. He was behind her doing the procedure.

I tried one last time to warn him. "Wait, wait, wait! You need to cover yourself." I said concerned over what I knew about to happen. Imagine a water balloon that is full of feces and gas and liquid that is just waiting to let go.

"Shut up!" He said again, raising his voice. "I know what I'm doing."

"Fine," I said, finally giving up.

Have you ever watched the old Loony Tunes cartoons? What happened next reminded me of a scene from one of those cartoons. Imagine you have a silhouette of a person standing against a wall, and the person gets sprayed with paint. When they walk away, you can still see the outline on the wall. Well, that's what happened with the senior resident, only instead of paint, it was fecal matter.

He immediately inserted the scope and had her colon untwisted in very short order, which literally caused an explosion.

Sometimes time seems to move very slowly. I saw what was happening as if it were in slow motion. I saw the shock and horror register on the senior resident's face as he reflexively tried to back up. "Noooo—" he cried through his mask. I could only hope that he had closed his mouth in time.

When it was over, I could see his silhouette on the floor and back wall. I could not tell from his facial expression what he was thinking, because his face was completely covered in feces, but I thought I could hazard a guess.

I turned my head away quickly, struggling not to laugh, but I needn't have worried about discretion. Turning on his heel he power walked from the room, leaving me to finish up with the patient.

We never spoke about what happened in the room that day, although word got around. In fact, for a while it became a bit of a joke among the other interns to start conversations with, "Oh, you think *you're* having a crappy day?"

Sometimes you just have to laugh.

CHAPTER 26

Medical Mission

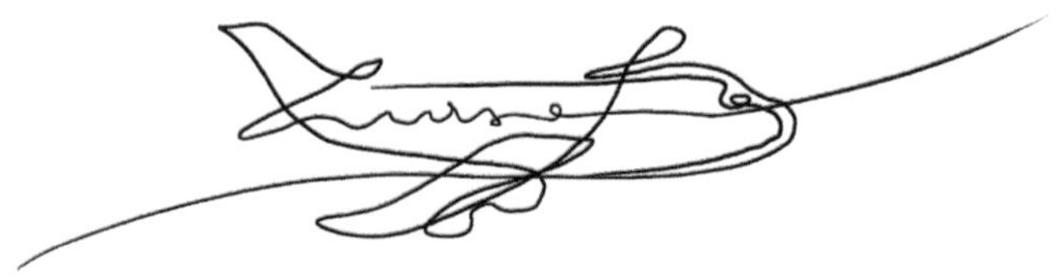

Over the years I have gone on a number of medical missions, treating patients in Palestine. I work with an American charitable organization, and they work through a busy, yet basic hospital set up there. On these neurosurgical missions, we bring donated equipment with us, and we see a lot of patients. We do as many surgeries as we safely can, but obviously there are some cases where the surgical requirements are too complex and require a more sophisticated hospital environment.

In some of these cases, I can only recommend more conservative treatment options, but sometimes the charity I work with is able to bring a patient who has more complex issues to the United States for treatment. One such case comes to mind; it involved a young girl named Sarah, who was about fourteen years old. Sarah was suffering from a debilitating spinal condition that, sadly, could not be repaired at that hospital. It bothered me not to be able to help this girl, who had such a sweet disposition, but the risk was too great given the circumstances. It was only by geography of birth that children like Sarah could not be helped. Had she been born in the US, she would have had access to much better medical care. This bothered me so much, that I approached the hospital where I worked in the US to discuss her case. The hospital agreed to let me do the surgery for free and to zero out their costs, and the charity paid to have the girl and her mother flown in. I of course was willing to volunteer my time free of charge, as was the anesthesiologist and other healthcare providers involved in her case.

When Sarah was flown out to see us in Southern California, she was accompanied by her mother, Nabila. We arranged for them to stay at a Ronald McDonald House, which is a place that families from out of town can stay at when a child is being treated in the hospital. When families have to travel to hospitals that are far from where they live to obtain treatment for their sick children, the costs of accommodation alone can be financially devastating. Charities such as the Ronald McDonald House help mitigate these costs and make it possible for families to stay together while their child is receiving treatment.

Sarah's surgery went well and although it was a complicated case, she did amazing. In fact, she only had to stay in the hospital for twenty-four hours. Within a week of Sarah's surgery, word had spread about her story, and several people in the area expressed an interest in wanting to help her family out. Their lives were difficult and people felt compassion for their plight. I was quite touched by the outpouring of support for Sarah and her mom. To me, it was a wonderful example of community collaboration and the kindness of the human spirit.

As soon as it was safe to do so, members of the community took Sarah and her mother to Disneyland, to the beach, and brought them sight-seeing. Sarah continued to improve and had no difficulty participating in these fun adventures. Both she and her mother had the time of their lives, and every time I saw them, they seemed to be laughing or smiling. We had them stay for about a month, so we could make sure Sarah's wounds were healing appropriately.

When Sarah and her mother flew back home, I felt happy with the knowledge that Sarah's chances of living a healthy, full life had been increased dramatically. About a year after they'd returned home, they sent me a video. In the video, Sarah and her mom said hello and thanked me and everyone else who had helped them. They reported that Sarah was doing great, that she was back to school, and finally back to just being a kid, doing the things that kids were supposed to do. Their video warmed my heart and brought tears to my eyes. Helping people on these missions is so incredibly rewarding. Every day I think about how fortunate we are, and it renews my determination to help improve the lives of others.

Looking back over my career thus far, I have acquired a wealth of stories, experiences, and memories; some of these are sad, others are interesting or inspiring, and some are downright funny. I try to learn something from every interaction to become a better person so that I can use the lessons learned to help others. I hope my book has inspired others to appreciate the human spirit, mind, body and soul.

ABOUT THE AUTHOR

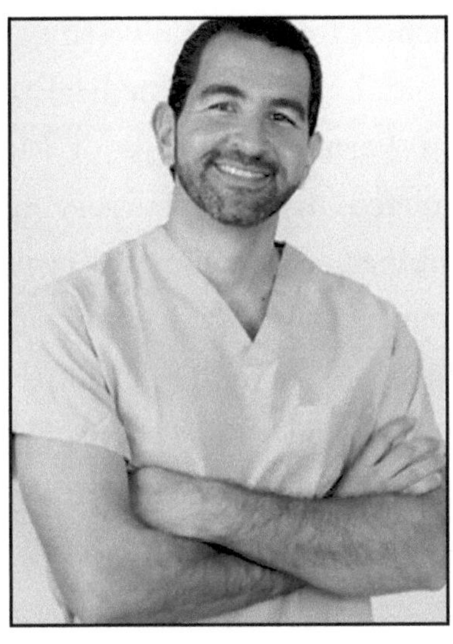

Burak Ozgur, MD is a neurosurgeon and Chief of Service for the Neurosurgical Spine Program at Hoag Hospital, Newport Beach. Dr. Ozgur is double board-certified by the American Board of Neurological Surgery and the American Board of Spine Surgery. He specializes in minimally invasive surgical techniques for common degenerative and complex disorders of the spine, including tumors, stenosis, and trauma. Dr. Ozgur also has a strong interest in stem cell research, spinal biomechanics, and innovative minimally invasive spine surgery development and research. He is helping to develop 3-D spine surgical navigation technology and the use of augmented reality in spine surgery. He received his undergraduate degree in biological sciences from the University of California, Irvine (UCI) and completed medical school at the University of Vermont, College of Medicine. Dr. Ozgur completed his neurosurgery residency, as well as a combined orthopedic surgery/neurosurgery spine fellowship, at the University of California, San Diego Medical Center. Dr. Ozgur has authored over 30 articles in peer-reviewed publications, has made over 130 presentations at various venues, has written nine book chapters, and recently published a surgical textbook, Minimally Invasive Spine Surgery: A Practical Guide to Anatomy and Techniques. Dr. Ozgur is also a member of the Society for Minimally Invasive Spine Surgery, AANS/CNS Spine Section, AANS, CNS, and the North American Spine Society. Dr. Ozgur also is the Founder and Director of ONE Brain and Spine Center in Irvine and Newport Beach

ozgurmd.com
Instagram @burakozgurmd

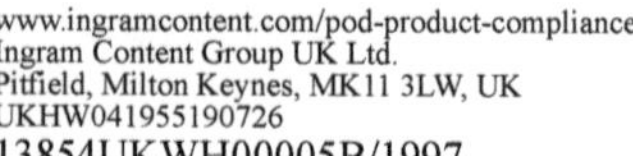

www.ingramcontent.com/pod-product-compliance
Ingram Content Group UK Ltd.
Pitfield, Milton Keynes, MK11 3LW, UK
UKHW041955190726
13854UKWH00005B/1997

9 798985 062755